ANTI-INFLAMM COOKBOOK FOR BEGINNERS:

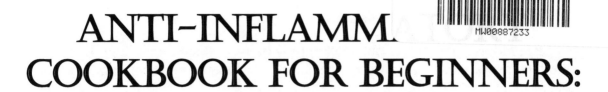

Follow Simple Dietary Guidelines to Boost Your Immune System, Reduce Inflammation, and Achieve Ideal Health by Improving Diet Habits, and Detoxing Your Body.

75-Day Meal Plan

by Duncan Hammond

Table of contents

INTRODUCTION

Inflammation: it's a word that has become all too common in our daily lives, often whispered in the corridors of doctors' offices, and splashed across health magazine headlines. Yet, the true impact of chronic inflammation on our bodies and minds remains a tale not entirely told.

So, what's the big deal about inflammation? At a fundamental level, inflammation is the body's innate response to injury or invasion by harmful agents. It's a crucial part of the immune system's defense mechanism, signaling the body to heal and repair damaged tissue. However, chronic inflammation is the silent intruder in your body's attic, contributing to a host of unwanted guests like arthritis, and heart disease, and even throwing your sugar levels into a frenzy.

The twist? You can evict this annoying intruder, and this book is your eviction notice. Now, before you think, "Ugh, another health guide?" – hold onto your hats. This isn't just another drop in the ocean of health guides that promise much and deliver little. It's the lighthouse guiding your ship safely to shore. The battle against this invisible foe is not just important; it's essential for reclaiming the quality of life that every individual deserves.

Picture this: You've got a buddy who's been through the wringer of inflammation. They've felt the burn, they've seen the swell, and they've come out the other side ready to spill the beans. Meet your author and ally, Dr. Duncan Hammond. He's lived the pain, embraced the struggle, and has now turned his victory into your roadmap for wellness. He's not just throwing science at you but mixing it with a bit of real-life grit.

The author has done the homework, diving deep into the research and teaming up with the pros in nutrition to create this guide. It's not just about understanding the tricky business of inflammation; it's packed with solid, doable tips to help you get a handle on it. Each chapter is infused with the latest findings from the fields of nutrition, immunology, and gastroenterology, ensuring that the recommendations are not just effective but also grounded in scientific evidence.

This isn't about wading through medical jargon or getting lost in the weeds of technical terms. No, this book is like a heart-to-heart with a friend who's seen it all, studied the science, chewed the fat with nutrition gurus, and is ready to lay it out plain and simple. This isn't just a cookbook; it's a companion on your journey to wellness.

But why this book, you might ask, in a world cluttered with health advice? What sets this book apart is its heart. The heart of someone who has walked the path of discomfort and emerged victorious on the other side. With each page, the author extends a hand, inviting you to join in the battle against the inflammation that besieges so many of us.

But here's the real secret sauce: every recipe in this book is a team effort. Dr. Hammond's nutritional know-how and his wife's culinary wizardry come together to make dishes that aren't just good for you—they're a delight for your taste buds, too. She's the chef with the knack for making healthy food taste like a treat, ensuring that every meal is a celebration of flavor.

Do you find yourself asking why you feel sluggish, why your joints ache, or why your digestive system seems to be in constant disarray? Are you tired of navigating through conflicting dietary advice, unsure of what truly works for your body? If that's something you're hoping to figure out, rest assured, that this book provides clarity amidst confusion, offering evidence-based, personalized guidance that respects your body's unique needs.

Did you know that the humble cinnamon you sprinkle on your latte has a secret identity? It's not just a spice; it's a powerhouse that can lower blood sugar levels and fight inflammation like a superhero in disguise.

Those processed snacks we all binge on during a Netflix marathon? They can trigger inflammation faster than you can say "just one more episode." It's like each chip is a tiny gremlin you're feeding after midnight, unleashing chaos in your body.

Now, don't get me started on sugar. That sweet, sweet crystal is practically inflammation's BFF. They hold hands and skip through your bloodstream, leaving a trail of inflammatory breadcrumbs that can lead to a witch's house of health woes.

But here's the kicker, the real shocker that might have you rethinking your whole pantry: some of the foods we've been told are 'healthy' could be undercover agents for Team Inflammation if your body doesn't agree with them.

So, what's a body to do with all these inflammatory insurgents lurking around every corner? That's where this book comes in. With every page turn, you'll uncover secrets to a lifestyle that doesn't just fight inflammation but dances on its grave. You'll learn to make food your ally – not the kind that says it'll help you move and then bails, but the kind that's with you lifting every box, every step of the way. With each recipe, you'll savor the flavor of healing, turning the act of eating from a mundane task into a delightful journey towards wellness.

So, are you ready to flip the script on inflammation? To wake up feeling like a superhero, rather than a character from "The Walking Dead"? If you're nodding your head (hopefully not too stiffly), then you're in the right place.

This book promises more than just improvement; it offers a transformation. Imagine waking up each day with more energy, less pain, and a brighter outlook on life. Picture a life where each meal brings you closer to the best version of yourself. This isn't a distant dream; it's a tangible reality that begins with the choices we make at the dining table. Now, stand at the threshold of change and peer into the future—a future where you are in control of your health, free from the constraints of chronic inflammation. It is more than a cookbook; it's a manifesto for a life reclaimed, a life full of energy, joy, and vitality.

Are you ready to take that step? To transform not just your diet, but your life? If the answer is a resounding "Yes," then let's begin this journey together.

Welcome to your new beginning!

Part one: Understanding Inflammation and the Healing Power of Food

CHAPTER 1: THE INFLAMMATION SPECTRUM AND ITS IMPACT ON HEALTH

Defining Inflammation: The Body's Response to Harm

Inflammation is not merely a symptom but a complex biological process involving the body's immune system. It's designed as a protective response to harmful stimuli, such as pathogens, damaged cells, or irritants, and it plays a vital role in the body's healing process. Understanding the science behind inflammation provides insight into how and why it occurs, enabling us to make informed decisions about managing it.

Inflammation begins when the immune system detects a threat to the body. This threat could be an invading microbe, plant pollen, a chemical, or even a physical injury like a cut or scrape. In response, the body's immune cells release various substances, including histamines, prostaglandins, and cytokines, which help to increase blood flow to the affected area. This increase in blood flow brings more immune cells to the site, facilitating the removal of harmful stimuli and the initiation of the healing process.

In the simplest terms, inflammation is your body's way of saying, "I've got this," when faced with anything it doesn't quite like, from injuries to infections. Think of it as the body's equivalent of posting a "Beware of Dog" sign, except the dog is your immune system, and the sign is swelling, redness, heat, and sometimes pain.

Acute vs. Chronic Inflammation

Acute Inflammation:

Inflammation is a word that often carries a negative connotation, conjuring images of redness, swelling, and pain. Indeed, it is the body's immediate response to an unwelcome event—a sprained ankle, a bee sting, or a bacterial invasion. This acute inflammatory response is critical for survival, a sign that your body's defense system is doing its job, rushing to protect you from harm and initiate he healing process. These symptoms are the result of the biological processes happening at the cellular level. For example, warmth and redness occur due to increased blood flow, while swelling results from the accumulation of fluid and immune cells in the tissue.

Literally. Without inflammation, injuries wouldn't heal, and infections could run rampant. Acute inflammation helps isolate affected areas, preventing invaders from traveling elsewhere in the body. So, while it might not feel great, it's a sign that your body's defense mechanisms are doing their job.

Chronic inflammation:

When the inflammation process persists, it becomes chronic. This can happen for several reasons: the initial cause of inflammation may not be resolved, the body may mistakenly target healthy tissues (as seen in autoimmune diseases), or a low-level response may continue due to chronic low-grade infections or ongoing exposure to a particular irritant. Unlike acute inflammation, chronic inflammation does not serve a protective or healing purpose. Instead, it can lead to tissue damage and contribute to the development of various diseases.

f inflammation had a social media status, it would be "It's complicated." Sometimes, it's the hero we all need, rushing in to save the day. Other times, it's like the friend who overstays their welcome, causing more problems than they solve.

Reasons for Inflammation

The reasons for inflammation are as diverse as the stimuli that trigger it. They can be categorized into external and internal causes:

External Causes: These include physical injuries, exposure to toxins, burns, frostbite, and foreign bodies like splinters or pathogens such as bacteria, viruses, and fungi.

Internal Causes: These can be more complex and include autoimmune reactions, where the body's immune system mistakenly attacks healthy cells, and the presence of chronic low-grade infections. Additionally, factors such as stress, obesity, and lifestyle choices (e.g., smoking, and alcohol consumption) can contribute to the maintenance of a chronic inflammatory state.

The Role of Diet and Lifestyle in Inflammation

The science behind inflammation underscores the significant impact of diet and lifestyle on our body's inflammatory responses. Certain foods, like processed sugars and unhealthy fats, can exacerbate inflammation, while others, such as omega-3 fatty acids found in fish and antioxidants present in fruits and vegetables, can help reduce it. Similarly, lifestyle choices such as regular physical activity, stress management, and avoiding smoking and excessive alcohol consumption can also play a crucial role in managing inflammation.

Understanding the biological mechanisms of inflammation highlights the importance of addressing both its causes and its effects. By integrating anti-inflammatory foods into our diet and making healthy lifestyle choices, we can support our body's natural defenses, reduce the risk of chronic inflammation, and promote overall health and well-being.

The Gut-Inflammation Axis: Exploring the Link

Our gut does more than just break down that cheeseburger from last night; it plays a crucial role in our immune response. This is thanks to the trillions of bacteria residing in the gut, collectively known as the microbiome. Think of it as a crowded city, where instead of people, you have bacteria, and instead of traffic jams, you have food particles and immune cells.

The gut microbiome is an incredibly diverse community of bacteria, viruses, fungi, and other microorganisms residing in our digestive tract. These microbes are not mere passengers; they play an essential role in digesting food, synthesizing nutrients, regulating the immune system, and protecting against pathogens. The balance of these microbial communities is critical for maintaining gut health and, by extension, our overall health.

The intestinal lining, or gut barrier, is another key player in the gut-inflammation nexus. This barrier is incredibly thin—just one cell layer separates the gut's interior from the rest of the body. Its integrity is vital in preventing unwanted substances from "leaking" into the bloodstream, which can trigger an immune response and inflammation. When this barrier is compromised, a condition known as "leaky gut" syndrome, it can lead to increased intestinal permeability, allowing toxins, undigested food particles, and bacteria to escape into the bloodstream and ignite inflammatory processes throughout the body.

A significant portion of the body's immune system resides in the gut, making it a critical battleground for fighting off pathogens and managing immune responses. A healthy, balanced gut microbiome promotes tolerance, preventing the immune system from overreacting to non-harmful antigens, which can lead to autoimmune diseases and chronic inflammation.

Dysbiosis, an imbalance in the gut microbiome, can lead to an increase in harmful bacteria and a decrease in beneficial ones, disrupting the gut barrier's integrity and immune function. This imbalance can set off a chain reaction, leading to chronic inflammation not just in the gut but throughout the entire body. Conditions such as inflammatory bowel disease (IBD), irritable bowel syndrome (IBS), and even non-digestive diseases like arthritis, diabetes, and heart disease have been linked to dysbiosis and gut inflammation.

Fact: Your Gut Has a Mind of Its Own

Scientifically known as the enteric nervous system, the gut's brain is in constant chatter with your actual brain, influencing everything from mood to inflammation. When this line of communication is clear, it's like having a smooth-running diplomatic channel. But when it gets crossed? That's when inflammation can spike, leading to a gut rebellion.

The good news is that by nurturing our gut health through diet, lifestyle, and potentially probiotics, we can influence our body's inflammatory response. A diet rich in fiber, fermented foods, and diverse plant-based foods can help foster a healthy microbiome, reinforcing the gut barrier and reducing the risk of inflammation-related disease

Prebiotics, Probiotics, and Diet: Strategies for a Healthy Gut

Prebiotics and probiotics emerge as the dynamic duo, working tirelessly to maintain order in the digestive tract.

Probiotics are live bacteria and yeasts that are beneficial for our digestive system. Often referred to as "good" or "friendly" bacteria, they help keep our gut healthy by enhancing the gut microbiome's diversity and functionality. They're like the skilled contractors you hire to renovate your home; they come in, assess the situation, and get to work fixing everything from leaky pipes (the gut barrier) to squeaky floors (digestive discomfort). Consuming probiotics can help restore the natural balance of the gut flora, which can be disrupted by factors such as antibiotics, poor diet, and stress.

Sources of probiotics include:

- Fermented foods like yogurt
- Kefir, sauerkraut, tempeh, and kimchi
- Supplements, for those who may need higher doses or specific strains

Probiotics work by enhancing mucosal immunity, strengthening the gut barrier, and modulating the body's immune response to prevent excessive inflammation.

While probiotics introduce beneficial bacteria into the gut, prebiotics serve as fuel for those bacteria to thrive. Prebiotics are a type of dietary fiber found in certain plants that human enzymes cannot digest. However, these fibers are fermented by the gut microbiota, promoting the growth and activity of beneficial bacteria.

Think of prebiotics as the dietary fiber that your body doesn't digest. Instead, they saunter through your digestive system, arriving in the colon like food trucks, ready to feed the hungry masses (your good bacteria). They're the ultimate support system, ensuring the local bacteria thrive and keep the neighborhood (your gut) in tip-top shape.

Dietary fiber from prebiotic-rich foods such as bananas, onions, garlic, leeks, asparagus, and artichokes is like the ultimate fertilizer for beneficial gut bacteria. Studies have shown that a diet high in prebiotics can increase the proliferation of good bacteria, which in turn can improve digestion, enhance mineral absorption, and even modulate the immune response.

Prebiotic-rich foods include:

- Garlic, onions, leeks, and shallots
- Asparagus, artichokes, and bananas
- Whole grains, such as barley, and oats
- Legumes, including lentils, chickpeas, and beans

Incorporating a variety of prebiotic foods into your diet supports a healthy microbiome, enhancing gut health and reducing inflammation.

Dietary Strategies for Gut Health

- **Diversity**: Eating a wide range of plant-based foods increases microbiome diversity, which is linked to better health.
- **Fiber**: High-fiber foods, beyond providing prebiotics, help regulate bowel movements and reduce the risk of gut-related diseases.
- **Moderation in Processed Foods**: Reducing intake of processed, high-sugar, and high-fat foods can decrease the prevalence of harmful bacteria that trigger inflammation.
- **Hydration**: Adequate water intake is essential for maintaining the mucosal lining of the intestines and supporting overall digestive health.

Adopting a diet that emphasizes prebiotics, probiotics, and overall nutritional balance is a powerful strategy for nurturing your gut health. By doing so, you not only support your digestive system but also contribute to a systemic reduction in inflammation, paving the way for improved health and vitality.

Inflammation's Role in Autoimmune Disorders

Autoimmune disorders occur when the immune system, the body's defense against invaders, mistakenly targets healthy cells, leading to a spectrum of diseases, each with unique symptoms but sharing a common inflammatory root. The National Institutes of Health (NIH) reports that up to 23.5 million Americans suffer from autoimmune diseases, with inflammation being a central feature of their pathology. From rheumatoid arthritis (RA) and lupus to multiple sclerosis (MS) and type 1 diabetes, these disorders share a common mechanism: the misdirected attack of the immune system, fueled by chronic inflammation.

Chronic inflammation in autoimmune diseases is not limited to specific areas of the body. It can have systemic effects, impacting a wide range of bodily functions and contributing to the development of comorbidities such as cardiovascular disease, increased susceptibility to infections, and metabolic syndrome. The systemic nature of this inflammation underscores the importance of managing it effectively to improve patient outcomes.

Research reveals that autoimmune diseases stem from a complex dance between genetics and environment, with inflammation as the lead partner. For instance, the presence of certain genes can increase susceptibility to autoimmune diseases, but environmental factors—such as infections, diet, and stress—can trigger the inflammatory response. This dual influence underscores the multifaceted nature of inflammation in autoimmune disorders.

Managing inflammation through lifestyle and dietary changes can significantly impact disease management and quality of life. An anti-inflammatory diet, rich in antioxidants, omega-3 fatty acids, and phytonutrients, can help dampen the inflammatory response. Regular physical activity, adequate sleep, stress management, and avoiding inflammatory triggers like smoking and excessive alcohol consumption are also crucial components of an integrated approach to managing autoimmune conditions.

Diet, Inflammation, and Heart Health: Making the Connection

The intricate link between diet, inflammation, and heart health is a critical piece of the puzzle in understanding overall wellness.

Scientific studies have consistently shown that chronic inflammation is a significant risk factor for cardiovascular diseases, including heart disease and stroke. For instance, the landmark Harvard Women's Health Study found that women with the highest levels of C-reactive protein (a marker for inflammation) were more than twice as likely to have a heart attack as those with the lowest levels. This finding underscores the silent but deadly role of inflammation in damaging blood vessels, leading to plaque formation and, ultimately, cardiovascular events.

Consider the contrasting stories of John and Maria. John's diet is heavy in processed foods, red meats, and sugary drinks—foods known to spike inflammatory markers in the body. By his mid-40s, John began experiencing high blood pressure and was diagnosed with early-stage heart disease, a direct consequence of his dietary choices fueling inflammation and harming his heart.

Maria, on the other hand, follows a Mediterranean diet, rich in fruits, vegetables, whole grains, and fish. At 52, her energy levels are high, her cholesterol levels are in check, and her heart is in excellent condition. Maria's diet, abundant in anti-inflammatory foods, has shielded her from the inflammation-driven heart issues that plague many of her peers.

Adopting an anti-inflammatory diet is a proactive step toward improving heart health. This diet emphasizes:

- **Fruits and Vegetables**: Rich in antioxidants and phytochemicals that reduce inflammation.

- **Whole Grains**: High in fiber, which can lower blood cholesterol levels and promote a healthy gut microbiome, indirectly reducing inflammation.
- **Lean Protein Sources**: Such as fish and legumes, which include anti-inflammatory omega-3 fatty acids and other nutrients.
- **Healthy Fats**: Found in nuts, seeds, avocados, and olive oil, these fats are essential for managing inflammation and supporting overall heart health.

Navigating Menopause: Inflammation and Hormonal Fluctuations

Menopause: it's not just hot flashes and mood swings. As women journey through this natural phase of life, they often find themselves battling an invisible foe: inflammation.

As estrogen levels take a rollercoaster ride during menopause, so does the body's inflammation response. Studies suggest that declining estrogen levels are linked to an increase in markers of inflammation, such as C-reactive protein (CRP). It's like Mother Nature decided that hot flashes weren't enough of a party and threw in inflammation for good measure.

Estrogen, prior to its decline during menopause, serves an essential function in regulating the immune system and maintaining control over inflammation. As estrogen levels diminish, the body experiences a significant loss in its anti-inflammatory defense mechanisms. This shift results in an increase in inflammatory responses, akin to losing a vital member of a protective team, thereby exposing the body to heightened levels of inflammation.

Example: The Tale of Two Joints

Consider the case of Sarah, who breezed through her forties with nary a joint pain. Enter menopause, and suddenly, she's wondering why her knees are auditioning for the role of "cranky old door hinges." This isn't uncommon, as many women experience an increase in joint pain and stiffness during menopause, a direct nod to the inflammation lurking behind the scenes.

While menopause might feel like a hormonal bonfire, there are ways to keep the inflammatory flames at bay:

- **Dietary Delights**: Embrace foods rich in omega-3 fatty acids, antioxidants, and phytoestrogens. It's time to befriend salmon, berries, and flaxseeds. Think of them as your dietary firefighters, ready to douse those inflammatory fires.
- **Move It to Lose It**: Regular exercise can help reduce inflammation and improve menopausal symptoms. Whether it's yoga, swimming, or chasing after grandkids, what's important is moving in a way that sparks joy, not joint pain.\

- **Stress Less**: Easier said than done, but managing stress through meditation, deep breathing, or a hobby can help keep inflammation in check. Remember, stressing about stress only leads to more stress. It's like a dog chasing its tail, only less cute.

How Reducing Inflammation Can Aid in Weight Management

Embarking on a weight management journey often feels like being a contestant on a reality show you didn't sign up for surprises around every corner, unexpected challenges, and the occasional desire to vote yourself off the island. However, amidst the calorie counting and exercise regimes, there's a less-talked-about contestant playing a stealthy game: inflammation. Let's delve into how tackling inflammation can be your secret strategy in winning the weight management battle.

Chronic inflammation, particularly, has been linked to obesity, acting both as a cause and a consequence of weight gain. The science is clear: fat cells, especially those in the abdomen, are not just inert storage units but active players that produce inflammatory markers, leading to a vicious cycle of weight gain and inflammation.

Studies have shown that overweight and obese individuals often have higher levels of C-reactive protein (CRP), a marker for inflammation in the body. This isn't just a coincidence; it's a sign of the body in distress, signaling that the inflammation might be fueling further weight gain.

Consider the story of Alex, who embarked on numerous diet plans to shed excess weight, all with little to no success. Frustrated and nearly ready to give up, Alex stumbled upon research highlighting the link between chronic inflammation and weight plateau. Motivated by this new insight, Alex revamped his diet to focus on anti-inflammatory foods, cutting back on sugar and processed meals while welcoming more whole grains, leafy greens, and omega-3-rich fish into his meals.

The transformation was remarkable. Not only did Alex start to see the scale move for the first time in years, but he also noticed a significant boost in his energy levels and a reduction in the joint pain he'd accepted as a normal part of aging. It was as if Alex had found the missing piece of his weight management puzzle, hidden in plain sight within his inflammation levels.

Strategies for Dousing the Inflammatory Flames

- **Eat the Rainbow**: Incorporating a variety of fruits and vegetables in your diet isn't just for show. Each color offers different anti-inflammatory benefits, making your plate a palette of health benefits.
- **Go for the Omega-3s**: Fatty fish like salmon and mackerel are like the firefighters of inflammation. They come in with their omega-3 fatty acids and help put out the inflammatory fires, aiding in weight management.

- **Spice It Up**: Turmeric and ginger aren't just for flavor; they're inflammation's natural enemies. Adding a little spice to your life can go a long way in managing both inflammation and weight.

In the grand scheme of weight management, addressing inflammation is like discovering a shortcut on a long hike. It might not cut out the journey entirely, but it certainly makes the trek more manageable and, dare we say, enjoyable. So, as you lace up your sneakers and prep your anti-inflammatory snacks, remember that every step toward reducing inflammation is a step toward a healthier, happier you.

CHAPTER 2: PERSONALIZING YOUR ANTI-INFLAMMATORY DIET

Bio-individuality and dietary reactions. Recognizing allergies and sensitivities

Bio-individuality refers to the concept that each of us has unique food and lifestyle needs. It's like saying we all have our own nutritional thumbprint. Scientifically, this uniqueness is due to variations in our metabolism, genetics, microbiome composition, and even environmental factors. It means that one person's food paradise can be another's digestive distress.

Allergies are like your immune system's over-the-top reaction to a food it mistakenly thinks is harmful. It's as if your body's defense system watches too much action TV and goes all out at the slightest hint of a threat. Food sensitivities, on the other hand, are more like a subtle drama, with symptoms that can be less immediate and more varied.

Learning to recognize your body's signals when it comes to food reactions is like being a detective in your own digestive whodunit. Keep an eye out for clues such as gastrointestinal upsets, skin changes, and energy dips. Remember, your body is always talking; you just have to listen.

Strategies for managing dietary reactions

- **Food Diaries**: Keep a log of what you eat and how you feel afterward. It's the nutritional equivalent of being a private eye on your own case.
- **Elimination Diets**: Temporarily remove suspected culprits from your diet and reintroduce them one at a time. It's like holding auditions to see which food gets the part of the villain.
- **Professional Testing**: Sometimes, you need to call in the experts for allergy testing. Think of them as the CSI of the food reaction world.

Understanding and accepting your body's unique dietary needs is the key to optimizing your health. It's about personalizing your plate to suit your script, not someone else's. So, celebrate your bio-individuality—customize your diet to your body's needs, and you'll be on your way to feeling like the star in your own health show.

Pro-Inflammatory vs. Anti-Inflammatory Foods

In the great coliseum of nutrition, there's a constant battle raging between pro-inflammatory and anti-inflammatory foods. One team is sneakily setting fires throughout your body, while the other is dousing the flames. Let's take a ringside seat to understand the players, their tactics, and how you can bet on the winning team.

Pro-Inflammatory Foods: The Flamethrowers

On the one side, we have pro-inflammatory foods; think of them as the culinary equivalent of fire starters. They're the processed meats, refined sugars, and trans fats that wage war on your body, raising inflammation levels and generally causing chaos like a bull in a china shop.

Scientifically speaking, pro-inflammatory foods can increase levels of inflammatory biomarkers like C-reactive protein (CRP). Eating a diet high in these foods is akin to continuously poking the bear that is your immune system, and you won't like it when it's angry.

Sugar and Refined Carbohydrates

Sugar, that sweet siren, lures us in with promises of immediate joy, only to betray us to our inflammatory foes. The same goes for its accomplice, refined carbohydrates - the white breads, pastas, and pastries that spike our blood sugar levels faster than you can say "insulin rush."

Studies have linked high intake of sugar and refined carbs to increased levels of inflammation, insulin resistance, and obesity. It's like throwing a fuel-soaked log onto an already raging fire

Trans Fats and Processed Foods

Trans fats are the outlaws of the fat world, created by adding hydrogen to vegetable oil, a process that could make even Dr. Frankenstein blush. These fats are found in many processed foods and have been linked to increased risk of heart disease, stroke, and, you guessed it, inflammation.

The FDA took a stand against trans fats, acknowledging the danger they pose and phasing them out of the food supply.

Dairy and Gluten

For some, dairy and gluten are the Bonnie and Clyde of digestion, often on the run from the law of gut health. While not everyone is sensitive to these, those with lactose intolerance or celiac disease know all too well the inflammatory havoc they can wreak.

Lactose intolerance affects around 65 percent of the human population, according to the National Institutes of Health. Celiac disease, meanwhile, is an autoimmune disorder where gluten leads to inflammation in the small intestines.

Gluten and dairy walked into a bar, and the immune system said, "Sorry, we don't serve your kind here."

Anti-Inflammatory Foods: Firefighters

On the other side are the anti-inflammatory foods, the hydrants and fire extinguishers of the food world. They're rich in omega-3 fatty acids, antioxidants, and polyphenols, ready to calm the flames and repair the damage.

Omega-3 Fatty Acids: Sources and Benefits

Omega-3s are the superheroes of the fat world, found gallantly in foods like salmon, flaxseeds, and walnuts. They work by reducing the production of molecules and substances linked to inflammation, such as eicosanoids and cytokines.

Antioxidants and Polyphenols

These are your body's rust protectors, shielding cells from damage. Found in colorful fruits and veggies, they're like a fresh coat of paint on a weathered fence, protecting it from the elements. Berries, green tea, and dark chocolate are all loaded with these protective compounds.

Spices and Herbs: Turmeric, Ginger, and Beyond

Spices are the special ops of the anti-inflammatory forces, with turmeric and ginger being the top agents. Curcumin in turmeric and gingerol in ginger act like elite commandos, sneaking into your cells and deactivating inflammatory pathways.

Incorporating Whole Foods: Vegetables, Fruits, Whole Grains, and Lean Proteins

Whole foods are the infantry, the foot soldiers of the anti-inflammatory army. They bring a diverse set of skills to the battle—fiber, vitamins, minerals—all of which are essential in maintaining your body's defenses.

Navigating Dining Out and Social Gatherings

Dining out and attending social gatherings can often feel like navigating a culinary minefield, especially when you're trying to eat healthily. But fear not, social butterflies and foodies alike; this chapter is your guide to handling these situations with grace, good humor, and a smidge of scientific savvy.

Eating out doesn't have to mean tossing your nutrition goals out the window. With a bit of strategy, you can enjoy the social scene without your diet becoming a cautionary tale.

A study published in the Journal of the American Academy of Nutrition and Dietetics found that meals consumed outside the home tend to be higher in calories, fat, and sodium. It's like restaurants are the food version of Las Vegas; what happens there can stay with you... around your waist.

I always advise you to preview the menu online before visiting. You will become a menu maestro, pre-selecting dishes that align with your anti-inflammatory diet, ensuring you can enjoy the social experience without the post-meal inflammation blues.

Bringing a healthy dish to share not only ensures you have something to eat, but it can also influence the food choices of others, according to social psychology. It's like being a health influencer, but instead of likes, you get nods of appreciation from fellow guests.

Navigating Alcohol at Social Events

Alcohol can be the Achilles' heel of many a well-intentioned dieter. The trick is moderation. Alcohol can be inflammatory, but if you choose to partake, opt for the least inflammatory options. Red wine, in moderation, is a good choice due to its resveratrol content, which has been associated with anti-inflammatory properties.

Moderation is key. Excessive alcohol consumption can lead to a leaky gut, which can exacerbate inflammation.

Fact: Alcohol can lower inhibitions, leading to less healthy food choices. It's like each drink whispers, "You know you want to eat those fries."

I often suggest following the 'water rule': alternate each glass of alcohol with a glass of water to stay hydrated and help moderate intake.

When it comes to social gatherings, planning is key. Eat a healthy snack before you go, so you don't arrive hungrier than a bear after hibernation. And when you're there, focus on the people more than the buffet. Socialize away from the food tables to avoid unconscious nibbling.

Mindful eating strategies are proven to help manage portion sizes. When you're engaged in conversation, you eat slower, which helps you recognize fullness cues.

CHAPTER 3: 10 SECRETS TO ELIMINATE INFLAMMATION

Welcome to a chapter that's not about keeping secrets, but about sharing the wisdom of ages—and a bit of scientific savvy—to quell the flames of inflammation. This is a practical, fact-filled guide for those seeking to understand and manage their body's inflammatory response, with a dash of humor to make the medicine go down more pleasantly.

Secret 1
Stress Less, Live More

Stress is like the unwanted seasoning in life's kitchen; it can make things go from flavorful to overbearing in a heartbeat. Keep stress levels low, and your body won't feel the need to sound the inflammation alarm.

High stress is linked to increased levels of the hormone cortisol, which can lead to systemic inflammation. Stress management techniques have been shown to decrease the production of pro-inflammatory cytokines, a type of signaling protein.

Did you know that chronic stress can shrink your brain? Studies have shown that prolonged stress can reduce gray matter in regions tied to emotion and physiological functions, which can have an inflammatory knock-on effect throughout the body.

If stress burned calories, we'd all be supermodels by now!

Studies indicate that stress-reduction interventions can lead to a 15-23% reduction in cortisol levels. Swap your late-night work emails for evening walks, find activities that cut stress and stick with them. Remember, a laugh a day keeps the inflammation at bay!

Secret 2
The Sleep Prescription

Skimping on sleep is like leaving your immune system on a never-ending night shift. It gets cranky, and it gets even—in the form of inflammation.

Sleep orchestrates a symphony of biological processes that fine-tune every aspect of your health. During deep sleep, the body enters a state of repair, restoring tissues and regulating the hormones that control inflammation, such as cortisol and adrenaline.

Shockingly, studies have found that individuals who consistently sleep less than six hours per night are at a significantly increased risk for chronic inflammation, with elevated levels of inflammatory markers like CRP (C-reactive protein) and IL-6 (interleukin-6).

Adults who get less than six hours of sleep per night have a 50% increase in the risk of viral infections and an increase in inflammatory diseases. Embrace the power of a pre-sleep ritual. Just as you wouldn't sprint into a wall and expect it to open, you can't leap from high activity into deep sleep without a transition. Dim the lights, avoid screens, and let your mind wind down with a book or meditation.

Secret 3
Gut Health

Your gut is the garden where health blossoms. Tend to it with prebiotics and probiotics, and watch your inflammation wilt away.

Emerging research suggests that the gut microbiome's influence extends beyond the gut itself, potentially affecting everything from mental health to the risk of diseases such as arthritis and heart disease.

A balanced gut microbiome is critical in maintaining the integrity of the gut barrier and regulating the immune system, thus controlling inflammation. People with a diversified gut microbiome have up to a 30% lower risk of inflammation-related illnesses.

Secret 4
Eat the Rainbow

Eating a variety of colorful, plant-based foods is like getting VIP access to nature's antioxidant party. Each pigment in these foods, from the deep purple of blueberries to the vibrant orange of carrots, carries unique phytonutrients that combat oxidative stress—a precursor to inflammation.

Each color in plant-based foods represents a different suite of phytonutrients, which are like the body's natural paintbrush against inflammation. The phytonutrients found in colorful fruits and vegetables can bind to and neutralize free radicals, rogue molecules that damage cells and increase inflammation. Diets rich in fruits and vegetables can lead to a 20-30% reduction in markers for inflammation.

Secret 5
Hydration is Holy

Water might just be the most underrated anti-inflammatory agent. Adequate hydration keeps every system in your body functioning optimally, flushing out potential inflammatory agents.

Cells rely on water to flush out toxins and carry nutrients. When dehydrated, your body is under stress, and cellular function is compromised, leading to an increase in inflammation.

It's not widely known that chronic dehydration can be as damaging to the kidneys as some diseases. Dehydrated tissues are breeding grounds for inflammation, with some studies showing that even mild dehydration can interfere with brain function, mood, and energy levels. Increasing water intake to the recommended 8 glasses a day can improve cellular hydration levels, potentially reducing inflammation by up to 21%.

Secret 6
Season with Purpose

Your spice rack holds more than just flavor; it's a pharmacy of anti-inflammatory agents. Spices such as turmeric, ginger, and cinnamon aren't just culinary; they're medicinal. Many spices have bioactive compounds with anti-inflammatory properties. Did you know that curcumin is so potent that it has been shown in some studies to match the effectiveness of some anti-inflammatory drugs, without the side effects? Regular consumption of anti-inflammatory spices has been associated with a decrease in the risk of inflammatory diseases by as much as 40%.

Secret 7
Move it to Improve it

Exercise can help reduce inflammation both directly and indirectly, by moderating weight and improving metabolic function. Engaging in regular physical activity initiates a fascinating biological cascade that, paradoxically, can both produce and reduce inflammatory markers. Initially, exercise increases oxidative stress and inflammation—this is the body's natural response to the exertion. However, this short-term spike is followed by a long-term decrease in baseline inflammation levels throughout the body.

Variety is the spice of life, and this holds true for exercise as well. Mixing up your workouts—cardio, strength training, flexibility exercises—ensures that all aspects of fitness are covered, and it keeps boredom at bay. Think of it as cross-training your immune system to be more efficient at managing inflammation.

Engaging in at least 150 minutes of moderate exercise per week can reduce inflammation markers by up to 35%.

Secret 8
Intermittent Fasting

Intermittent fasting (IF) is not just a dietary trend; it's a time-honored tradition with a modern twist that's catching the eyes of scientists and health enthusiasts alike.

Intermittent fasting can activate pathways in your body that reduce inflammation and improve metabolic health. During fasting periods, your body shifts from using glucose as its primary fuel source to using fatty acids and their by-products, called ketones. This switch can reduce inflammation, improve insulin sensitivity, and even promote better brain health.

Begin with the less rigorous 16:8 method, fasting for 16 hours and eating during an 8-hour window. This approach can ease your body into the fasting process and still yield significant anti-inflammatory benefits. Studies have found that intermittent fasting can reduce markers of inflammation, such as CRP, by up to 50% in some individuals. That's a significant drop, rivaling the effects of certain anti-inflammatory medications

Secret 9
Allergen Alert

Allergens are like those uninvited party crashers that can turn your body's immune system into an overprotective bouncer, causing inflammation when they show up. They can trigger an unnecessary inflammatory response that could otherwise be avoided with the right knowledge and vigilance.

When your body encounters an allergen, it responds by releasing antibodies—specifically, IgE antibodies—which in turn signal for the release of histamine and other chemicals, leading to an inflammatory response. If you suspect certain foods or environmental factors are causing inflammation, consider an elimination diet or allergy testing. Start by removing the suspected allergen from your diet or environment for a few weeks and monitor how you feel. Then, reintroduce the item and note any changes in symptoms.

Secret 10
Yoga

Yoga is the chill zone for your immune system. The practice of yoga, steeped in thousands of years of history, is more than just a series of stretches and poses—it's a full-body diplomatic negotiation for peace, influencing everything from muscle tone to mental health, and yes, even inflammation.

Yoga goes beyond physical flexibility; it engages the parasympathetic nervous system (PNS), which is responsible for the 'rest and digest' responses in the body. Activation of the PNS through yoga can reduce the levels of stress hormones in the body, which are known contributors to inflammation. A study published in the Journal of Behavioral Medicine found that yoga practitioners had lower levels of inflammatory markers compared to non-practitioners, suggesting that regular practice could have a substantial effect on reducing inflammation.

Incorporate a variety of yoga styles into your routine. While gentle forms like Hatha can calm the system, more active styles like Vinyasa can improve circulation and physical health, both contributing to lower inflammation.

Part Two: Anti-inflammatory Cookbook

CHAPTER 4: BREAKFAST AND BRUNCH RECIPES

TURMERIC GINGER OATMEAL

INGREDIENTS
- 1 cup rolled oats
- 2 cups water or plant-based milk
- 1 teaspoon turmeric powder
- 1/2 teaspoon ginger powder
- A pinch of black pepper (to enhance turmeric absorption)
- 1 tablespoon maple syrup or honey
- 1/4 cup chopped walnuts
- 1 banana, sliced
- egg noodles
- 3/4 cup sour cream, or to taste

Preparation time:	Cook time:	Total time:
5 min	5 min	10 min

DIRECTIONS
Cook: In a saucepan, bring the oats and water/milk to a boil, then reduce heat to simmer. Add turmeric, ginger, and black pepper.
Stir: Continue to cook, stirring occasionally, until the oats are soft and creamy.
Sweeten: Remove from heat and stir in maple syrup or honey.
Serve: Top with chopped walnuts and banana slices. Enjoy warm.

Nutritional Breakdown (Estimated per serving): Calories: 300-400 kcal, Protein: 8-10 g, Fat: 4-6 g (Saturated Fat: 1-2 g), Carbs: 60-70 g (Dietary Fiber: 8-10 g, Sugars: 10-15 g)

SWEET POTATO AND KALE HASH

INGREDIENTS

- 1 large sweet potato, peeled and diced
- 2 cups kale, chopped
- 1/2 red onion, diced
- 2 tablespoons olive oil
- Salt and pepper to taste
- 1/2 teaspoon smoked paprika

Preparation time:	Cook time:	Total time:
10 min	15 min	25 min

DIRECTIONS

Sauté: In a large skillet, heat olive oil over medium heat. Add diced sweet potato and onion; cook until the potatoes are tender.

Add Kale: Stir in the kale until wilted. Season with salt, pepper, and smoked paprika.

Serve: Enjoy warm as a nutrient-dense, anti-inflammatory breakfast.

Nutritional Breakdown (Estimated per serving): Calories: 250-300 kcal, Protein: 4-6 g, Fat: 14-16 g (Saturated Fat: 2-3 g), Carbs: 30-35 g (Dietary Fiber: 5-7 g, Sugars: 7-9 g)

SMOKED SALMON AND AVOCADO OMELET

INGREDIENTS

- 2 large eggs
- 1 tablespoon almond milk or water
- Salt and pepper, to taste
- 1/2 tablespoon olive oil
- 2 ounces smoked salmon, sliced
- 1/2 ripe avocado, sliced
- 1 tablespoon chopped fresh chives or dill, plus extra for garnish
- 1/4 teaspoon ground turmeric
- Optional: a sprinkle of red pepper flakes for extra anti-inflammatory benefits and a bit of heat

Preparation time:	Cook time:	Total time:
5 min	10 min	15 min

DIRECTIONS

Prepare Eggs: In a bowl, whisk together the eggs, almond milk (or water), turmeric, salt, and pepper until light and frothy. Adding turmeric not only adds a beautiful color but also provides anti-inflammatory benefits.

Cook Omelette: Heat the olive oil in a non-stick skillet over medium heat. Pour in the egg mixture, tilting the pan to spread it evenly. Cook for 1-2 minutes until the eggs are set on the bottom.

Add Fillings: Before the omelet is fully set, arrange the smoked salmon slices and avocado slices over half of the omelet. Sprinkle with chopped chives or dill, and add red pepper flakes if using.

Fold and Finish: Carefully fold the other half of the omelet over the fillings. Let it cook for another 2-3 minutes until the eggs are fully set and the filling is heated through.

Serve: Carefully slide the omelet onto a plate. Garnish with additional herbs for a fresh touch. Serve immediately.

Nutritional Breakdown (Estimated per serving): Calories: 350 kcal, Protein: 25 g, Fat: 26 g (Saturated Fat: 6 g), Carbs: 8 g (Dietary Fiber: 5 g, Sugars: 1 g)

CHIA SEED PUDDING WITH MANGO

INGREDIENTS
- 1/4 cup chia seeds
- 1 cup coconut milk
- 1 tablespoon maple syrup or honey
- 1/2 teaspoon vanilla extract
- 1 ripe mango, peeled and cubed

Preparation time:	Cook time:	Total time:
5 min	0 min	5 min

DIRECTIONS
Mix: In a bowl, combine chia seeds, coconut milk, maple syrup, and vanilla extract. Stir well.
Refrigerate: Cover and refrigerate overnight or for at least 6 hours.
Serve: Once set, stir the pudding, then top with mango cubes before serving.

BLUEBERRY ALMOND PROTEIN PANCAKES

INGREDIENTS
- 1 cup gluten-free all-purpose flour
- 1/2 cup almond flour
- 1 tablespoon baking powder
- 1/4 teaspoon salt
- 1 cup almond milk
- 1 egg
- 1 tablespoon maple syrup
- 1 teaspoon vanilla extract
- 1/2 cup blueberries (fresh or frozen)
- 1 tablespoon coconut oil (for cooking)

Preparation time:	Cook time:	Total time:
10 min	10 min	20 min

DIRECTIONS

Mix Dry Ingredients: In a large bowl, combine gluten-free all-purpose flour, almond flour, baking powder, and salt.

Add Wet Ingredients: In another bowl, whisk together almond milk, egg, maple syrup, and vanilla extract. Pour the wet ingredients into the dry ingredients and stir until just combined.

Fold in Blueberries: Gently fold in the blueberries.

Cook: Heat a non-stick skillet or griddle over medium heat and brush with coconut oil. Pour 1/4 cup batter for each pancake and cook until bubbles form on the surface, then flip and cook until golden brown.

Serve: Enjoy warm, topped with extra blueberries and a drizzle of maple syrup if desired.

Nutritional Breakdown (Estimated per serving): Calories: 300-400 kcal, Protein: 15-20 g, Fat: 10-15 g (Saturated Fat: 1-2 g), Carbs: 40-50 g (Dietary Fiber: 5-7 g, Sugars: 10-15 g)

SWEET POTATO HASH WITH SPINACH AND EGGS

INGREDIENTS

- 2 medium sweet potatoes, peeled and diced
- 2 tablespoons olive oil
- 1/2 teaspoon paprika
- Salt and pepper to taste
- 2 cups fresh spinach
- 4 large eggs
- Optional: avocado slices and fresh herbs for garnish

Preparation time:	Cook time:	Total time:
10 min	20 min	30 min

DIRECTIONS

Cook Sweet Potatoes: Heat olive oil over medium heat in a large skillet. Add the sweet potatoes, paprika, salt, and pepper. Cook, stirring occasionally, until the sweet potatoes are tender and slightly crispy, about 15 minutes.
Add Spinach: Stir in the spinach until wilted, about 2 minutes.
Cook Eggs: Make four wells in the hash and crack an egg into each. Cover and cook until the eggs are set to your liking, about 4-6 minutes.
Serve: Garnish with avocado slices and fresh herbs if desired. Enjoy warm.

Nutritional Breakdown (Estimated per serving): Calories: 300-400 kcal, Protein: 12-15 g, Fat: 15-20 g (Saturated Fat: 3-5 g), Carbs: 35-45 g (Dietary Fiber: 6-8 g, Sugars: 10-12 g)

AVOCADO TOAST WITH POACHED EGG

INGREDIENTS
- 2 slices gluten-free bread
- 1 ripe avocado
- Salt and pepper to taste
- 1 large egg
- Optional garnishes: red pepper flakes, fresh herbs (such as cilantro or parsley)

Preparation time:	Cook time:	Total time:
5 min	5 min	10 min

DIRECTIONS
Poach Egg: Bring a small pot of water to a simmer. Crack the egg into a cup, then gently slide it into the simmering water. Cook for 3-4 minutes for a soft poached egg or until your desired doneness. Remove with a slotted spoon and drain on a paper towel.

Toast Bread: While the egg is poaching, toast the gluten-free bread slices to your liking.

Mash Avocado: In a bowl, mash the avocado with a fork. Season with salt and pepper.

Assemble: Spread the mashed avocado evenly onto the toasted bread slices. Place the poached egg on top of one slice. Add optional garnishes such as red pepper flakes or fresh herbs if desired.

Serve: Enjoy immediately for a simple yet nutritious and satisfying breakfast.

Nutritional Breakdown (Estimated per serving): Calories: 300-350 kcal, Protein: 12-15 g, Fat: 20-25 g (Saturated Fat: 3-5 g), Carbs: 15-20 g (Dietary Fiber: 7-10 g, Sugars: 2-3 g)

MEDITERRANEAN SHAKSHUKA

INGREDIENTS

- 2 tablespoons olive oil
- 1 large onion, thinly sliced
- 2 garlic cloves, minced
- 1 bell pepper, sliced
- 2 cups chopped tomatoes (fresh or canned)
- 1 teaspoon paprika
- 1 teaspoon cumin
- 1/2 teaspoon turmeric
- Salt and pepper to taste
- 4-6 large eggs
- Optional for serving: avocado slices, fresh cilantro, gluten-free bread or pita

Preparation time:	Cook time:	Total time:
10 min	20 min	30 min

DIRECTIONS

Sauté Veggies: Heat the olive oil over medium heat in a large skillet. Add the onion and bell pepper, sautéing until softened. Stir in the garlic and cook for another minute.

Add Tomatoes & Spices: Add the chopped tomatoes, paprika, cumin, turmeric, salt, and pepper. Simmer for 10-15 minutes until the sauce has thickened.

Cook Eggs: Make wells in the sauce and crack an egg into each. Cover and cook over low heat until the eggs are set to your preference.

Serve: Garnish with avocado slices and fresh cilantro. Serve with gluten-free bread or pita.

Nutritional Breakdown (Estimated per serving): Calories: 250-300 kcal, Protein: 12-15 g, Fat: 15-18 g (Saturated Fat: 3-4 g), Carbs: 20-25 g (Dietary Fiber: 4-5 g, Sugars: 8-10 g)

SWEET POTATO AND BLACK BEAN BURRITOS

INGREDIENTS
- 2 medium sweet potatoes, peeled and diced
- 1 tablespoon olive oil
- 1 teaspoon cumin
- 1/2 teaspoon smoked paprika
- Salt and pepper to taste
- 1 can (15 oz) black beans, rinsed and drained
- 1/2 cup corn (fresh or frozen)
- 4 gluten-free tortillas
- 1 avocado, sliced
- Optional garnishes: lime wedges, cilantro, dairy-free sour cream

Preparation time:	Cook time:	Total time:
15 min	30 min	45 min

DIRECTIONS
Roast Sweet Potatoes: Preheat the oven to 400°F (200°C). Toss the sweet potatoes with olive oil, cumin, paprika, salt, and pepper. Roast for 20-25 minutes until tender.

Warm Beans & Corn: In a pan, warm the black beans and corn with a pinch of salt and pepper.

Assemble Burritos: Warm the gluten-free tortillas according to package instructions. Divide the sweet potato mixture, black beans, and corn among the tortillas. Add avocado slices.

Serve: Roll up the burritos and serve with lime wedges, cilantro, and dairy-free sour cream if desired.

Nutritional Breakdown (Estimated per serving): Calories: 350-400 kcal, Protein: 10-12 g, Fat: 10-12 g (Saturated Fat: 2-3 g), Carbs: 60-65 g (Dietary Fiber: 10-12 g, Sugars: 5-6 g)

QUINOA SALAD WITH LEMON-TAHINI DRESSING

INGREDIENTS
- 1 cup quinoa (rinsed)
- 2 cups water
- 1 cup cherry tomatoes, halved
- 1 cucumber, diced
- 1/4 cup red onion, finely chopped
- 1/4 cup parsley, chopped
- 2 tablespoons tahini
- Juice of 1 lemon
- 2 tablespoons olive oil
- Salt and pepper to taste

Preparation time:	Cook time:	Total time:
15 min	20 min	35 min

DIRECTIONS

Cook Quinoa: In a saucepan, bring quinoa and water to a boil. Reduce heat, cover, and simmer for 15 minutes or until quinoa is fluffy and water is absorbed. Let it cool slightly.

Prepare Dressing: In a small bowl, whisk together tahini, lemon juice, olive oil, salt, and pepper until smooth. Adjust seasoning to taste, and add a little water if the dressing is too thick.

Combine Salad Ingredients: In a large bowl, combine the cooked quinoa, cherry tomatoes, cucumber, red onion, and parsley. Toss to mix evenly.

Dress the Salad: Pour the lemon-tahini dressing over the salad and toss again until everything is well coated.

Serve: Serve the salad at room temperature or chilled. It can be enjoyed independently or as a side dish to a larger meal. Optional garnishes include additional parsley, lemon wedges, or a sprinkle of sesame seeds.

Nutritional Breakdown (Estimated per serving): Calories: 300-350 kcal, Protein: 8-10 g, Fat: 18-20 g (Saturated Fat: 2-3 g), Carbs: 30-35 g (Dietary Fiber: 5-6 g, Sugars: 3-4 g)

CHAPTER 5: LUNCH AND DINNER RECIPES

BAKED SALMON WITH AVOCADO SALSA

INGREDIENTS
- 4 salmon fillets (about 6 ounces each)
- 2 tablespoons olive oil
- Salt and pepper to taste
- 1 large avocado, diced
- 1/2 cup cherry tomatoes, quartered
- 1/4 cup red onion, finely chopped
- 1/4 cup cilantro, chopped
- Juice of 1 lime
- 1 tablespoon extra virgin olive oil
- 1 garlic clove, minced
- 1 teaspoon of fresh jalapeño, finely chopped (optional for extra heat)

Preparation time:	Cook time:	Total time:
15 min	20 min	35 min

DIRECTIONS

Preheat Oven & Prepare Salmon: Preheat your oven to 375°F (190°C). Line a baking sheet with parchment paper. Place the salmon fillets on the prepared sheet and drizzle with 2 tablespoons of olive oil. Season generously with salt and pepper. Bake for about 15-20 minutes, or until the salmon is cooked through and flakes easily with a fork.

Make Avocado Salsa: While the salmon is baking, prepare the avocado salsa. In a medium bowl, combine the diced avocado, quartered cherry tomatoes, finely chopped red onion, chopped cilantro, lime juice, extra virgin olive oil, minced garlic, and jalapeño if using. Gently toss to combine. Season with salt and pepper to taste.

Assemble & Serve: Remove the salmon from the oven and cool slightly once the salmon is done. Serve each salmon fillet topped with a generous portion of avocado salsa.

Nutritional Breakdown (Estimated per serving): Calories: 400-450 kcal, Protein: 25-30 g, Fat: 25-30 g (Saturated Fat: 4-5 g), Carbs: 20-25 g (Dietary Fiber: 7-8 g, Sugars: 3-4 g)

TURMERIC CHICKEN AND QUINOA

INGREDIENTS

- 4 chicken breasts, boneless and skinless
- 1 teaspoon turmeric
- 1 teaspoon garlic powder
- Salt and pepper to taste
- 1 tablespoon olive oil
- 1 cup quinoa, rinsed
- 2 cups chicken broth or water
- 1 cup spinach, chopped
- 1/4 cup almonds, sliced

Preparation time:	Cook time:	Total time:
10 min	20 min	30 min

DIRECTIONS

Season Chicken: Combine turmeric, garlic powder, salt, and pepper. Rub the mixture over the chicken breasts.

Cook Quinoa: In a saucepan, bring quinoa and broth to a boil. Reduce heat, cover, and simmer for 15 minutes. Stir in spinach and let sit until wilted.

Grill Chicken: While quinoa cooks, heat olive oil in a skillet over medium heat. Add chicken and cook for 6-7 minutes per side or until fully cooked.

Serve: Slice chicken and serve over a bed of quinoa and spinach. Garnish with sliced almonds.

Nutritional Breakdown (Estimated per serving): Calories: 350-400 kcal, Protein: 30-35 g, Fat: 10-15 g (Saturated Fat: 2-3 g), Carbs: 40-45 g (Dietary Fiber: 5-6 g, Sugars: 2-3 g)

VEGGIE STIR-FRY

INGREDIENTS
- 2 tablespoons sesame oil
- 1 bell pepper, sliced
- 1 cup broccoli florets
- 1/2 cup carrots, julienned
- 1/2 cup snap peas
- 2 garlic cloves, minced
- 1 tablespoon ginger, grated
- 2 tablespoons soy sauce (or tamari for a gluten-free option)
- 1 tablespoon maple syrup
- 1 tablespoon apple cider vinegar
- Optional: sesame seeds, green onions for garnish

Preparation time:	Cook time:	Total time:
15 min	10 min	25 min

DIRECTIONS
Sauté Veggies: In a large skillet or wok, heat sesame oil over medium-high heat. Add bell pepper, broccoli, carrots, and snap peas. Stir-fry for 5-7 minutes until vegetables are tender but still crisp.

Add Flavour: Stir in garlic and ginger, cooking for another minute. Add soy sauce, maple syrup, and apple cider vinegar. Stir well to combine and coat the vegetables.

Serve: Serve the stir-fry hot, garnished with sesame seeds and chopped green onions if desired.

Nutritional Breakdown (Estimated per serving): Calories: 200-250 kcal, Protein: 6-8 g, Fat: 10-15 g (Saturated Fat: 1-2 g), Carbs: 25-30 g (Dietary Fiber: 5-7 g, Sugars: 10-12 g)

LEMON GARLIC BAKED COD WITH ASPARAGUS

INGREDIENTS

- 4 cod fillets (6 ounces each)
- 2 tablespoons olive oil
- 4 garlic cloves, minced
- Juice and zest of 1 lemon
- Salt and pepper to taste
- 1 bunch asparagus, trimmed
- Optional garnish: lemon slices and fresh parsley

Preparation time:	Cook time:	Total time:
10 min	20 min	30 min

DIRECTIONS

Prepare Asparagus: Toss asparagus with 1 tablespoon olive oil, salt, and pepper. Arrange in a single layer on one side of the prepared baking sheet.

Season Cod: Place cod fillets on the other side of the baking sheet. Drizzle with the remaining olive oil and sprinkle with minced garlic, lemon juice, zest, salt, and pepper.

Bake: Bake in the preheated oven for 15-20 minutes, or until the cod flakes easily with a fork and asparagus is tender.

Serve: Garnish with lemon slices and fresh parsley before serving.

Nutritional Breakdown (Estimated per serving): Calories: 200-250 kcal, Protein: 20-25 g, Fat: 10-12 g (Saturated Fat: 1-2 g), Carbs: 5-10 g (Dietary Fiber: 2-3 g, Sugars: 2-3 g)

KALE AND QUINOA SALAD WITH ORANGE-TAHINI DRESSING

INGREDIENTS
- 1 cup quinoa, rinsed
- 2 cups water
- 4 cups kale, stems removed and leaves chopped
- 1/2 cup sliced almonds
- 1/4 cup dried cranberries
  For the dressing:
- 3 tablespoons tahini
- Juice of 1 orange
- 1 tablespoon apple cider vinegar
- 1 tablespoon maple syrup
- Salt and pepper to taste

Preparation time:	Cook time:	Total time:
15 min	15 min	30 min

DIRECTIONS

Cook Quinoa: In a medium saucepan, bring quinoa and water to a boil. Reduce heat, cover, and simmer for about 15 minutes or until water is absorbed. Let it cool.

Blanch Kale: Briefly blanch the kale in boiling water, then rinse under cold water. Squeeze out excess moisture.

Prepare Dressing: Whisk together tahini, orange juice, apple cider vinegar, maple syrup, salt, and pepper in a small bowl until smooth.

Assemble Salad: In a large bowl, combine cooled quinoa, blanched kale, sliced almonds, and dried cranberries. Drizzle with dressing and toss to combine.

Serve: Enjoy this nutrient-rich salad as a refreshing lunch or dinner.

Nutritional Breakdown (Estimated per serving):
Calories: 300-350 kcal, Protein: 10-12 g, Fat: 15-18 g (Saturated Fat: 2-3 g), Carbs: 40-45 g (Dietary Fiber: 8-10 g, Sugars: 5-7 g)

GINGER TURMERIC CHICKEN STIR-FRY

INGREDIENTS

- 2 tablespoons coconut oil
- 1 pound chicken breast, thinly sliced
- 2 cloves garlic, minced
- 1 inch ginger, grated
- 1 teaspoon turmeric
- 1 bell pepper, sliced
- 1 cup broccoli florets
- 1/2 cup snap peas
- 2 tablespoons soy sauce or tamari
- 1 tablespoon honey
- Optional: sesame seeds and green onions for garnish

Preparation time:	Cook time:	Total time:
10 min	20 min	30 min

DIRECTIONS

Cook Chicken: Heat coconut oil in a large skillet over medium-high heat. Add chicken and cook until browned and cooked through. Remove chicken and set aside.

Sauté Vegetables: In the same skillet, add garlic, ginger, and turmeric. Cook for about 1 minute until fragrant. Add bell pepper, broccoli, and snap peas. Stir-fry until vegetables are just tender.

Combine: Return chicken to the skillet. Add soy sauce and honey. Stir well to combine all ingredients and cook for another 2-3 minutes.

Serve: Garnish with sesame seeds and green onions if desired. Serve hot.

Nutritional Breakdown (Estimated per serving): Calories: 250-300 kcal, Protein: 25-30 g, Fat: 10-12 g (Saturated Fat: 1-2 g), Carbs: 15-20 g (Dietary Fiber: 3-4 g, Sugars: 5-6 g)

ROASTED BEET AND GOAT CHEESE SALAD

INGREDIENTS
- 4 medium beets, peeled and cubed
- 2 tablespoons olive oil
- Salt and pepper to taste
- 4 cups mixed greens
- 1/2 cup goat cheese, crumbled
- 1/4 cup walnuts, chopped

For the dressing:

- 3 tablespoons balsamic vinegar
- 1 tablespoon honey
- 1/3 cup olive oil
- Salt and pepper to taste

Preparation time:	Cook time:	Total time:
15 min	45 min	1 hour

DIRECTIONS

Roast Beets: Preheat oven to 400°F (200°C). Toss beets with olive oil, salt, and pepper. Spread on a baking sheet and roast for 45 minutes or until tender and slightly caramelized, stirring occasionally.

Prepare Dressing: In a small bowl, whisk together balsamic vinegar, honey, olive oil, salt, and pepper until well combined and emulsified.

Assemble Salad: In a large bowl, toss the mixed greens with half of the dressing. Divide the greens among plates.

Add Beets and Toppings: Top each salad with roasted beets, crumbled goat cheese, and chopped walnuts. Drizzle with the remaining dressing.

Serve: Enjoy this colorful and nutritious salad as a light lunch or a side dish at dinner. The combination of sweet roasted beets, tangy goat cheese, and crunchy walnuts makes for a delightful and anti-inflammatory meal.

Nutritional Breakdown (Estimated per serving): Calories: 200-250 kcal, Protein: 6-8 g, Fat: 15-18 g (Saturated Fat: 5-6 g), Carbs: 15-20 g (Dietary Fiber: 4-5 g, Sugars: 10-12 g)

SPICY SWEET POTATO AND BLACK BEAN CHILI

INGREDIENTS
- 2 tablespoons olive oil
- 1 large onion, diced
- 2 cloves garlic, minced
- 2 medium sweet potatoes, peeled and cubed
- 1 red bell pepper, diced
- 2 cans (15 oz each) black beans, drained and rinsed
- 1 can (28 oz) diced tomatoes
- 2 tablespoons chili powder
- 1 teaspoon cumin
- 1/2 teaspoon smoked paprika
- Salt and pepper to taste
- 2 cups vegetable broth
- Optional garnishes: avocado slices, cilantro, lime wedges

Preparation time:	Cook time:	Total time:
15 min	30 min	45 min

DIRECTIONS

Sauté Onion and Garlic: In a large pot, heat olive oil over medium heat. Add onion and garlic, sautéing until softened.

Add Sweet Potatoes and Spices: Stir sweet potatoes, bell pepper, chili powder, cumin, and smoked paprika. Cook for 2-3 minutes, stirring frequently.

Combine and Simmer: Add black beans, diced tomatoes (with their juice), and vegetable broth. Bring to a boil, then reduce heat and simmer for 20-25 minutes or until the sweet potatoes are tender.

Serve: If desired, ladle the chili into bowls and garnish with avocado slices, cilantro, and lime sweet roasted beets, tangy goat cheese, and crunchy walnuts makes for a delightful and anti-inflammatory meal.

Nutritional Breakdown (Estimated per serving): Calories: 300-350 kcal, Protein: 12-15 g, Fat: 5-8 g (Saturated Fat: 1-2 g), Carbs: 60-65 g (Dietary Fiber: 15-18 g, Sugars: 10-12 g)

SALMON PASTA WITH SUN-DRIED TOMATOES

INGREDIENTS

- 8 ounces whole wheat pasta (or any preferred pasta)
- 2 salmon fillets (about 6 ounces each)
- 2 tablespoons olive oil
- Salt and pepper to taste
- 1/2 cup sun-dried tomatoes, chopped
- 2 cloves garlic, minced
- 1 cup spinach, fresh
- 1/2 cup coconut milk
- 1/4 cup low-sodium vegetable broth (or chicken broth)
- 1 tablespoon lemon juice
- 1 teaspoon lemon zest
- 1/4 cup basil, chopped (for garnish)
- Red pepper flakes (optional, for heat)

Preparation time:	Cook time:	Total time:
15 min	20 min	35 min

DIRECTIONS

Cook Pasta: Cook the pasta according to package instructions in a large pot of salted boiling water until al dente. Drain and set aside, reserving 1 cup of the pasta water for later.

Prepare Salmon: While the pasta is cooking, season the salmon fillets with salt and pepper. Heat 1 tablespoon of olive oil in a skillet over medium heat. Add the salmon, skin-side down, and cook for 4-5 minutes on each side or until cooked through and easily flaked with a fork. Transfer the salmon to a plate, flake it into bite-sized pieces with a fork, and set aside.

Sauté Garlic and Sun-Dried Tomatoes: In the same skillet, add the remaining olive oil, sun-dried tomatoes, and garlic. Sauté for 2-3 minutes.

Add Spinach and Liquids: Add the spinach to the skillet and cook until it begins to wilt. Stir in the coconut milk, vegetable broth, lemon juice, and lemon zest. Bring the mixture to a simmer.

Combine Pasta and Salmon: Add the cooked pasta to the skillet, tossing it to coat it in the creamy sauce. If the sauce is too thick, add some reserved pasta water until you reach your desired consistency. Gently fold in the flaked salmon, not breaking the pieces too much.

Serve: Divide the pasta among plates. Garnish with chopped basil and red pepper flakes if using. Serve immediately.

Nutritional Breakdown (Estimated per serving):
Calories: 550-600 kcal, Protein: 30-35 g, Fat: 20-25 g (Saturated Fat: 5-6 g, Omega-3s: High), Carbs: 65-70 g (Dietary Fiber: 4-5 g, Sugars: 5-6 g)

VEGAN COCONUT CHICKPEA CURRY

INGREDIENTS
- 1 tablespoon coconut oil
- 1 large onion, finely chopped
- 3 cloves garlic, minced
- 1 tablespoon fresh ginger, grated
- 1 tablespoon turmeric powder
- 1 teaspoon cumin powder
- 1 teaspoon coriander powder
- 1/2 teaspoon cayenne pepper (adjust according to taste)
- 1 can (14 oz) chickpeas, drained and rinsed
- 1 can (14 oz) diced tomatoes
- 1 can (14 oz) coconut milk (full-fat for creaminess)
- 1 large sweet potato, cubed
- 1 red bell pepper, sliced
- Salt to taste
- Fresh cilantro, chopped (for garnish)
- Juice of 1 lime

Preparation time:	Cook time:	Total time:
10 min	25 min	35 min

DIRECTIONS
Sauté Aromatics: Heat coconut oil in a large skillet or saucepan over medium heat. Add the onion and sauté until soft and translucent, about 5 minutes. Add the garlic and ginger, and sauté for another minute until fragrant.

Add Spices: Stir in the turmeric, cumin, coriander, and cayenne pepper. Cook for about 1 minute, stirring constantly to prevent the spices from burning.

Combine Ingredients: Add the chickpeas, diced tomatoes (with their juice), coconut milk, sweet potato, and red bell pepper to the skillet. Stir well to combine all the ingredients. Season with salt to taste.

Simmer: Bring the curry to a boil, then reduce the heat to low. Cover and let it simmer for about 20 minutes until the sweet potato is tender and the flavors melded together.

Final Touches: Once the curry is done, turn off the heat and stir in the lime juice. Adjust seasoning if necessary.

Serve: Ladle the curry into bowls and garnish with chopped cilantro. Serve hot, accompanied by cooked rice or naan bread if desired.

Nutritional Breakdown (Estimated per serving):
Calories: 350-400 kcal, Protein: 10-12 g, Fat: 18-20 g (Saturated Fat: 12-14 g), Carbs: 40-45 g (Dietary Fiber: 9-11 g, Sugars: 8-9 g)

BUDDHA BOWL

INGREDIENTS
- 1 cup quinoa, rinsed
- 1 sweet potato, peeled and cubed
- 1 beet, peeled and cubed
- 2 cups kale, chopped
- 1 tablespoon olive oil
- Salt and pepper to taste
- 1 avocado, sliced
- 1/2 cup red cabbage, shredded
- 1/4 cup pumpkin seeds

For the dressing:
- 3 tablespoons tahini
- 1 tablespoon maple syrup
- Juice of 1 lemon
- Salt and water to adjust consistency, chopped (for garnish)
- Juice of 1 lime

Preparation time:	Cook time:	Total time:
20 min	30 min	50 min

DIRECTIONS

Cook Quinoa: In a saucepan, combine quinoa with 2 cups of water. Bring to a boil, then reduce heat, cover, and simmer for 15 minutes or until water is absorbed. Fluff with a fork.

Roast Vegetables: Preheat oven to 400°F (200°C). Toss sweet potato and beet cubes with olive oil, salt, and pepper. Spread on a baking sheet and roast for 25-30 minutes, until tender.

Sauté Kale: Heat a pan over medium heat, add kale with a splash of water, and sauté until wilted, about 5 minutes. Season with salt and pepper.

Prepare Dressing: Whisk together tahini, maple syrup, lemon juice, salt, and water (as needed) until smooth.

Assemble Buddha Bowls: Divide quinoa among bowls. Top with roasted sweet potatoes, beets, sautéed kale, avocado slices, shredded red cabbage, and pumpkin seeds. Drizzle with tahini dressing.

Serve: Enjoy this nourishing bowl packed with various textures and flavors, along with anti-inflammatory benefits.

Nutritional Breakdown (Estimated per serving):
Calories: 400-450 kcal, Protein: 12-15 g, Fat: 20-25 g (Saturated Fat: 3-4 g), Carbs: 50-55 g (Dietary Fiber: 10-12 g, Sugars: 8-10 g)

SPICY LENTIL AND SWEET POTATO STEW

INGREDIENTS
- 1 tablespoon olive oil
- 1 onion, chopped
- 2 garlic cloves, minced
- 1 teaspoon ground cumin
- 1/2 teaspoon smoked paprika
- 1/4 teaspoon cayenne pepper (adjust to taste)
- 1 sweet potato, peeled and cubed
- 1 cup lentils (rinsed)
- 1 can (14.5 oz) diced tomatoes
- 4 cups vegetable broth
- Salt and pepper to taste
- Optional garnishes: fresh cilantro, dollop of dairy-free yogurt

Preparation time:	Cook time:	Total time:
10 min	40 min	50 min

DIRECTIONS
Sauté Onion and Garlic: In a large pot, heat olive oil over medium heat. Add onion and garlic, cooking until soft and translucent.

Add Spices: Stir in cumin, smoked paprika, and cayenne pepper. Cook for another minute until fragrant.

Add Main Ingredients: Add sweet potatoes, lentils, diced tomatoes (with their juice), and vegetable broth. Bring to a boil, then reduce heat and simmer for 30-35 minutes or until the lentils and sweet potatoes are tender.

Season and Serve: Season the stew with salt and pepper to taste. Serve hot, garnished with fresh cilantro and a dollop of yogurt if desired.

Nutritional Breakdown (Estimated per serving):
Calories: 300-350 kcal, Protein: 15-18 g, Fat: 5-8 g (Saturated Fat: 1-2 g), Carbs: 60-65 g (Dietary Fiber: 15-18 g, Sugars: 12-14 g)

GINGER-LIME TOFU WITH BROCCOLI STIR-FRY

INGREDIENTS

- 1 block (14 ounces) of firm tofu, pressed and cubed
- 2 tablespoons soy sauce (low sodium)
- 1 tablespoon grated ginger
- Juice of 2 limes
- 1 tablespoon honey or maple syrup
- 2 tablespoons olive oil
- 2 cups broccoli florets
- 1 red bell pepper, sliced
- 1 carrot, julienned
- 2 garlic cloves, minced
- 1 tablespoon sesame seeds

Preparation time:	Cook time:	Total time:
15 min	20 min	35 min

DIRECTIONS

Marinate Tofu: In a bowl, combine tofu cubes with soy sauce, ginger, lime juice, and honey. Marinate for at least 30 minutes.

Stir-Fry Vegetables: Heat 1 tablespoon olive oil in a large pan over medium-high heat. Add broccoli, bell pepper, and carrot. Stir-fry for 5-7 minutes until vegetables are tender-crisp. Add garlic and stir-fry for another minute. Remove vegetables from the pan and set aside.

Cook Tofu: In the same pan, add the remaining 1 tablespoon of olive oil. Add marinated tofu and cook until golden brown on all sides, about 8-10 minutes.

Combine & Serve: Return the vegetables to the pan with the tofu. Toss to combine. Sprinkle with sesame seeds and serve immediately.

Nutritional Breakdown (Estimated per serving):
Calories: 300-350 kcal, Protein: 18-23 g, Fat: 10-15 g (Saturated Fat: 1-2 g), Carbs: 30-35 g (Dietary Fiber: 8-9 g, Sugars: 5-6 g)

CHAPTER 6: VEGETARIAN MENU

TURMERIC QUINOA WITH ROASTED VEGETABLES

INGREDIENTS
- 1 cup quinoa, rinsed
- 2 cups vegetable broth
- 1 teaspoon turmeric powder
- 1 sweet potato, cubed
- 1 red onion, sliced
- 2 cups Brussels sprouts, halved
- 2 tablespoons olive oil
- Salt and pepper to taste
- 1/4 cup chopped almonds
- 1/4 cup dried cranberries

Preparation time:	Cook time:	Total time:
15 min	25 min	40 min

DIRECTIONS

Cook Quinoa: In a pot, combine quinoa, vegetable broth, and turmeric. Bring to a boil, then reduce heat, cover, and simmer for 15 minutes or until quinoa is fluffy.
Roast Vegetables: Preheat oven to 425°F (220°C). Toss sweet potato, onion, and Brussels sprouts with olive oil, salt, and pepper. Spread on a baking sheet and roast for 20-25 minutes until tender and caramelized.
Combine & Serve: Mix cooked quinoa with roasted vegetables. Top with chopped almonds and dried cranberries before serving.

Nutritional Breakdown (Estimated per serving):
Calories: 320 kcal, Protein: 10 g, Fat: 14 g (Saturated Fat: 2 g), Carbs: 42 g (Dietary Fiber: 7 g, Sugars: 8 g)

SPICY BLACK BEAN AND SWEET POTATO TACOS

INGREDIENTS

- 2 sweet potatoes, peeled and cubed
- 1 can (15 ounces) black beans, drained and rinsed
- 1 tablespoon olive oil
- 1 teaspoon cumin
- 1/2 teaspoon smoked paprika
- 1/4 teaspoon chili powder
- Salt and pepper to taste
- 8 small corn tortillas
- 1 avocado, sliced
- 1/4 cup fresh cilantro, chopped
- Lime wedges for serving

Preparation time:	Cook time:	Total time:
20 min	30 min	50 min

DIRECTIONS

Roast Sweet Potatoes: Preheat oven to 425°F (220°C). Toss sweet potatoes with half the olive oil, cumin, smoked paprika, chili powder, salt, and pepper. Spread on a baking sheet and roast for 25 minutes, until tender.

Prepare Black Beans: Heat the remaining olive oil over medium heat. Add black beans and cook for 5 minutes or until heated through. Lightly mash the beans with a fork.

Assemble Tacos: Warm tortillas according to package instructions. Divide the sweet potatoes and black beans among the tortillas. Top with avocado slices and cilantro.

Serve: Offer lime wedges on the side for squeezing over tacos.

Nutritional Breakdown (Estimated per serving):
Calories: 280 kcal, Protein: 9 g, Fat: 7 g (Saturated Fat: 1 g), Carbs: 48 g (Dietary Fiber: 11 g, Sugars: 9 g)

MOZZARELLA, BASIL & ZUCCHINI FRITTATA

INGREDIENTS
- 8 large eggs, preferably omega-3 enriched
- 1 tablespoon extra virgin olive oil
- 2 medium zucchinis, thinly sliced
- 1 small onion, finely chopped
- 2 cloves garlic, minced
- 1/2 cup fresh basil leaves, chopped
- 1/2 cup dairy-free mozzarella cheese, shredded
- Salt (Himalayan pink salt recommended) and pepper to taste
- Optional: 1/4 teaspoon turmeric powder

Preparation time:	Cook time:	Total time:
10 min	35 min	45 min

DIRECTIONS

Preheat the Oven: Preheat your oven to 375°F (190°C) to ensure it's ready for baking.

Sauté the Vegetables: Heat the olive oil in a large ovenproof skillet over medium heat. Add the onion and garlic, and cook until they're soft and fragrant about 2-3 minutes. Incorporate the sliced zucchini and cook until just tender, which should take about 5 minutes. If you're using turmeric for an extra anti-inflammatory boost, sprinkle it over the vegetables now and mix well.

Prepare the Egg Mixture: Whisk the eggs thoroughly in a separate large bowl. Mix in the chopped basil and a pinch of salt and pepper to enhance the flavors.

Combine the Ingredients: Distribute the sautéed zucchini evenly across the bottom of the skillet. Gently pour the egg mixture over the zucchini, ensuring an even spread. Sprinkle the dairy-free mozzarella cheese on top for a creamy texture.

Cook on Stove: Allow the mixture to cook over medium heat for 2-3 minutes until the edges start to set.

Bake: Transfer the skillet into your preheated oven. Bake for 20-25 minutes, or until the frittata is fully set and the cheese has melted and turned slightly golden.

Serve: Let the frittata cool once out of the oven for a few minutes. Slice it into portions and serve warm for a delicious meal.

Nutritional Breakdown (Estimated per serving):
Calories: 350 kcal, Protein: 12 g, Fat: 10 g (Saturated Fat: 2 g), Carbs: 60 g (Dietary Fiber: 5 g, Sugars: 4 g)

ZUCCHINI NOODLES WITH AVOCADO PESTO

INGREDIENTS
- 4 large zucchinis, spiralized
- 1 ripe avocado
- 1/2 cup fresh basil leaves
- 1/4 cup pine nuts
- 2 tablespoons lemon juice
- 1 garlic clove
- Salt and pepper to taste
- Cherry tomatoes for garnish

Preparation time:	Cook time:	Total time:
15 min	0 min	15 min

DIRECTIONS
Make Avocado Pesto: In a food processor, blend avocado, basil, pine nuts, lemon juice, and garlic until smooth. Season with salt and pepper.
Prepare Zucchini Noodles: Place spiralized zucchini in a large bowl.
Combine & Serve: Toss zucchini noodles with avocado pesto until well coated. Serve topped with cherry tomatoes.

Nutritional Breakdown (Estimated per serving):
Calories: 220 kcal, Protein: 4 g, Fat: 18 g
(Saturated Fat: 3 g), Carbs: 14 g (Dietary Fiber: 7 g, Sugars: 3 g)

CHICKPEA AND KALE SALAD WITH LEMON-TAHINI DRESSING

INGREDIENTS

- 2 cans (15 ounces each) chickpeas, drained and rinsed
- 4 cups kale, chopped
- 1/2 red onion, thinly sliced
- 1/2 cup cherry tomatoes, halved
- 1/4 cup tahini
- 2 tablespoons lemon juice
- 1 garlic clove, minced
- 2 tablespoons water
- Salt and pepper to taste
- 1/4 cup pumpkin seeds

Preparation time:	Cook time:	Total time:
15 min	0 min	15 min

DIRECTIONS

Prepare Salad: In a large bowl, combine chickpeas, kale, red onion, and cherry tomatoes.

Make Dressing: In a small bowl, whisk together tahini, lemon juice, minced garlic, and water until smooth. Season with salt and pepper.

Combine & Serve: Pour dressing over the salad and toss to coat evenly. Sprinkle pumpkin seeds on top before serving.

Nutritional Breakdown (Estimated per serving):
Calories: 310 kcal, Protein: 9 g, Fat: 18 g (Saturated Fat: 2.5 g), Carbs: 32 g (Dietary Fiber: 9 g, Sugars: 5 g)

LENTIL STUFFED BELL PEPPERS

INGREDIENTS

- 4 large bell peppers, tops cut off and seeds removed
- 1 cup lentils, rinsed
- 2 cups vegetable broth
- 1 tablespoon olive oil
- 1 onion, finely chopped
- 2 garlic cloves, minced
- 1 carrot, diced
- 1 teaspoon cumin
- 1 teaspoon paprika
- Salt and pepper to taste
- 1 cup cooked rice (optional, for added bulk)
- 1/2 cup tomato sauce
- 1/4 cup fresh parsley, chopped

Preparation time:	Cook time:	Total time:
20 min	40 min	60 min

DIRECTIONS

Cook Lentils: In a medium saucepan, combine lentils and vegetable broth. Bring to a boil, then reduce heat and simmer covered until lentils are tender about 25-30 minutes. Drain any excess liquid.

Preheat Oven: Preheat your oven to 375°F (190°C).

Sauté Vegetables: While lentils cook, heat olive oil in a pan over medium heat. Add onion, garlic, and carrot. Cook until the vegetables are softened, about 5-7 minutes. Stir in cumin, paprika, salt, and pepper.

Combine Filling: Mix cooked lentils, sautéed vegetables, rice (if using), and tomato sauce in a bowl. Adjust seasoning as needed.

Stuff Peppers: Fill each bell pepper with the lentil mixture. Place the stuffed peppers upright in a baking dish. Add a small amount of water to the bottom of the dish (about 1/4 inch) to prevent sticking and help the peppers steam.

Bake: Cover the dish with foil and bake for about 30-40 minutes, or until the peppers are tender and the filling is heated through.

Serve: Garnish with fresh parsley before serving.

Nutritional Breakdown (Estimated per serving): Calories: 290 kcal, Protein: 14 g, Fat: 5 g (Saturated Fat: 1 g), Carbs: 50 g (Dietary Fiber: 13 g, Sugars: 9 g)

CHAPTER 7: SALADS AND SOUPS

AVOCADO AND SPINACH SALAD WITH BERRIES

INGREDIENTS
- 4 cups baby spinach
- 1 ripe avocado, diced
- 1 cup mixed berries (strawberries, blueberries, raspberries)
- 1/4 cup walnuts, chopped
- 2 tablespoons chia seeds
    For the dressing:
- 3 tablespoons extra virgin olive oil
- 1 tablespoon apple cider vinegar
- 1 teaspoon honey (or maple syrup for vegan option)
- Salt and pepper to taste

Preparation time:	Cook time:	Total time:
10 min	10 min	20 min

DIRECTIONS

Prepare the Salad: In a large bowl, combine the spinach, diced avocado, mixed berries, walnuts, and chia seeds.
Make the Dressing: Whisk together the olive oil, apple cider vinegar, honey, salt, and pepper in a small bowl.
Toss and Serve: Drizzle the dressing over the salad and gently toss to combine. Serve immediately for the freshest taste.

Nutritional Breakdown (Estimated per serving):
Calories: 220 kcal, Protein: 4 g, Fat: 18 g (Saturated Fat: 2.5 g), Carbs: 15 g (Dietary Fiber: 7 g, Sugars: 5 g)

CAESAR SALAD

INGREDIENTS
- 4 cups romaine lettuce, chopped
- 1 ripe avocado, diced
- 1/2 cup cherry tomatoes, halved
- 1/4 cup pumpkin seeds
- 2 tablespoons hemp seeds

  For the dressing:
- 3 tablespoons extra virgin olive oil
- 1 tablespoon lemon juice
- 1 teaspoon Dijon mustard
- 1 garlic clove, minced
- 1 teaspoon anchovy paste (optional; can omit for a vegetarian version)
- Salt and pepper to taste
- 1 tablespoon of dairy-free cheese

Preparation time:	Cook time:	Total time:
10 min	10 min	20 min

DIRECTIONS

Prepare the Salad: In a large bowl, combine the chopped romaine lettuce, diced avocado, cherry tomatoes, pumpkin seeds, and hemp seeds.

Make the Dressing: In a small bowl, whisk together the olive oil, lemon juice, Dijon mustard, minced garlic, anchovy paste (if using), salt, and pepper. Stir in the dairy-free cheese until well combined.

Toss and Serve: Drizzle the dressing over the salad and gently toss to combine. Ensure everything is evenly coated with the dressing. Serve immediately for the best flavor and texture.

Nutritional Breakdown (Estimated per serving): Calories: 250 kcal, Protein: 6 g, Fat: 20 g (Saturated Fat: 3 g), Carbs: 12 g (Dietary Fiber: 5 g, Sugars: 3 g)

CUCUMBER AND DILL SALAD WITH LEMON DRESSING

INGREDIENTS
- 2 large cucumbers, thinly sliced
- 1/4 red onion, thinly sliced
- 1/4 cup fresh dill, chopped
  For the dressing:
- 3 tablespoons extra virgin olive oil
- 2 tablespoons lemon juice
- 1 teaspoon honey (or maple syrup for vegan option)
- Salt and pepper to taste

Preparation time:	Cook time:	Total time:
10 min	10 min	20 min

DIRECTIONS
Prepare the Salad: In a large bowl, combine the sliced cucumbers, red onion, and fresh dill.
Mix the Dressing: In a small bowl, whisk together the olive oil, lemon juice, honey, salt, and pepper until well combined.
Combine: Pour the dressing over the cucumber mixture and toss gently to coat.
Chill and Serve: For the best flavor, let the salad chill in the refrigerator for about 30 minutes before serving.

Nutritional Breakdown (Estimated per serving):
Calories: 120 kcal, Protein: 2 g, Fat: 9 g (Saturated Fat: 1.5 g), Carbs: 9 g (Dietary Fiber: 2 g, Sugars: 4 g)

BROCCOLI AND ALMOND SALAD WITH GINGER DRESSING

INGREDIENTS
- 4 cups broccoli florets, raw or lightly steamed and cooled
- 1/2 cup sliced almonds, toasted
- 1/4 cup dried cranberries
  For the dressing:
- 1/4 cup extra virgin olive oil
- 2 tablespoons apple cider vinegar
- 1 tablespoon fresh ginger, grated
- 1 teaspoon honey (or maple syrup for vegan option)
- Salt and pepper to taste

Preparation time:	Cook time:	Total time:
15 min	0 min	15 min

DIRECTIONS

Prepare the Salad: In a large bowl, combine the broccoli florets, toasted sliced almonds, and dried cranberries.

Whisk the Dressing: In a small bowl, whisk together the olive oil, apple cider vinegar, grated ginger, honey, salt, and pepper until smooth.

Dress the Salad: Pour the ginger dressing over the broccoli mixture and toss to coat evenly.

Serve: Let the salad sit for at least 10 minutes before serving to allow the flavors to meld.

Nutritional Breakdown (Estimated per serving):
Calories: 235 kcal, Protein: 7 g, Fat: 18 g
(Saturated Fat: 2 g), Carbs: 15 g (Dietary Fiber: 6 g, Sugars: 4 g)

SWEET POTATO AND BLACK BEAN SALAD WITH LIME-CILANTRO VINAIGRETTE

INGREDIENTS

- 2 medium sweet potatoes, peeled and cubed
- 1 tablespoon olive oil
- Salt and pepper to taste
- 1 can (15 ounces) black beans, drained and rinsed
- 1 red bell pepper, diced
- 1/2 red onion, finely chopped
- 1/4 cup fresh cilantro, chopped

    For the Lime-Cilantro Vinaigrette:

- 1/4 cup extra virgin olive oil
- Juice of 2 limes
- 1 garlic clove, minced
- 2 tablespoons chopped fresh cilantro
- 1 teaspoon honey (or maple syrup for vegan option)
- Salt and pepper to taste

Preparation time:	Cook time:	Total time:
20 min	25 min	45 min

DIRECTIONS

Roast Sweet Potatoes: Preheat oven to 425°F (220°C). Toss the cubed sweet potatoes with olive oil, salt, and pepper. Spread on a baking sheet and roast for 25 minutes or until tender and slightly caramelized, stirring halfway through.

Prepare the Vinaigrette: In a small bowl, whisk together the olive oil, lime juice, minced garlic, chopped cilantro, honey, salt, and pepper. Adjust seasoning to taste.

Combine the Salad: In a large bowl, combine the roasted sweet potatoes, black beans, diced red bell pepper, red onion, and fresh cilantro. Drizzle with the lime-cilantro vinaigrette and toss gently to combine.

Serve: This salad can be served warm, at room temperature, or chilled. It's perfect as a stand-alone meal or as a side dish.

Nutritional Breakdown (Estimated per serving): Calories: 300 kcal, Protein: 8 g, Fat: 10 g (Saturated Fat: 1.5 g), Carbs: 48 g (Dietary Fiber: 11 g, Sugars: 8 g)

BUTTERNUT SQUASH SOUP WITH COCONUT MILK

INGREDIENTS
- 1 butternut squash, peeled, seeded, and cubed
- 1 tablespoon olive oil
- 1 onion, diced
- 2 garlic cloves, minced
- 4 cups vegetable broth
- 1 can (14 ounces) coconut milk
- 1 teaspoon curry powder
- Salt and pepper to taste
- Pumpkin seeds for garnish

Preparation time:	Cook time:	Total time:
20 min	30 min	50 min

DIRECTIONS
Sauté Vegetables: In a large pot, heat olive oil over medium heat. Add onion and garlic, cooking until softened.
Cook Squash: Add butternut squash, vegetable broth, and curry powder to the pot. Bring to a boil, reduce heat, and simmer until squash is tender, about 20 minutes.
Blend Soup: Using an immersion blender or standing blender, puree the soup until smooth. Stir in coconut milk and season with salt and pepper.
Serve: Warm the soup before serving, garnished with pumpkin seeds.

Nutritional Breakdown (Estimated per serving): Calories: 250 kcal, Protein: 3 g, Fat: 12 g (Saturated Fat: 9 g), Carbs: 35 g (Dietary Fiber: 5 g, Sugars: 8 g)

BROCCOLI AND TURMERIC SOUP

INGREDIENTS

- 1 butternut squash, peeled, seeded, and cubed
- 1 tablespoon olive oil
- 1 onion, diced
- 2 garlic cloves, minced
- 4 cups vegetable broth
- 1 can (14 ounces) coconut milk
- 1 teaspoon curry powder
- Salt and pepper to taste
- Pumpkin seeds for garnish

Preparation time:	Cook time:	Total time:
10 min	20 min	30 min

DIRECTIONS

Sauté Aromatics: In a large pot, heat the olive oil over medium heat. Add the onion and garlic, sautéing until they are soft and translucent.

Add Turmeric and Broccoli: Stir in the fresh turmeric, cooking for about a minute until fragrant. Add the broccoli florets and vegetable broth. Season with salt and pepper.

Simmer: Bring the soup to a boil, then reduce heat and let it simmer until the broccoli is tender, about 15 minutes.

Blend and Serve: Use an immersion blender to puree the soup until smooth. Stir in coconut milk for a creamier texture, if desired. Serve the soup garnished with pumpkin seeds for added texture and nutrients.

Nutritional Breakdown (Estimated per serving): Calories: 210 kcal, Protein: 6 g, Fat: 12 g (Saturated Fat: 1.5 g), Carbs: 22 g (Dietary Fiber: 5 g, Sugars: 5 g)

RED LENTIL AND SPINACH SOUP

INGREDIENTS
- 2 tablespoons olive oil
- 1 onion, diced
- 2 garlic cloves, minced
- 1 cup red lentils, rinsed
- 4 cups vegetable broth
- 2 teaspoons ground cumin
- 4 cups fresh spinach, roughly chopped
- Salt and pepper to taste
- Lemon wedges for serving

Preparation time:	Cook time:	Total time:
10 min	25 min	35 min

DIRECTIONS

Cook Onions and Garlic: In a large pot, heat olive oil over medium heat. Add the onion and garlic, cooking until the onion is translucent.

Add Lentils and Broth: Stir in the red lentils, vegetable broth, and ground cumin. Bring the mixture to a boil, then reduce heat and simmer until the lentils are tender about 20 minutes.

Add Spinach: Stir in the chopped spinach until it wilts in the soup, which will take just a few minutes.

Season and Serve: Season the soup with salt and pepper to taste. Serve hot with a wedge of lemon on the side, allowing guests to add a fresh squeeze of lemon juice for a bright flavor.

Nutritional Breakdown (Estimated per serving): Calories: 250 kcal, Protein: 15 g, Fat: 4 g (Saturated Fat: 0.5 g), Carbs: 40 g (Dietary Fiber: 10 g, Sugars: 3 g)

BUTTERNUT SQUASH AND APPLE SOUP

INGREDIENTS
- 2 tablespoons olive oil
- 1 onion, chopped
- 2 garlic cloves, minced
- 1 butternut squash, peeled, seeded, and cubed
- 2 apples, peeled, cored and chopped
- 4 cups vegetable broth
- 1 teaspoon ground cinnamon
- 1/2 teaspoon ground nutmeg
- Salt and pepper to taste
- Roasted pumpkin seeds for garnish

Preparation time:	Cook time:	Total time:
20 min	40 min	60 min

DIRECTIONS
Sauté Onion and Garlic: Heat olive oil in a large pot over medium heat. Add the onion and garlic, sautéing until they become soft and translucent.

Add Squash and Apples: Incorporate the butternut squash and apples into the pot, stirring to combine with the onion and garlic.

Simmer Soup: Pour the vegetable broth and season the mixture with cinnamon, nutmeg, salt, and pepper. Bring to a boil, lower the heat, and simmer until the squash and apples are tender, about 30 minutes.

Puree and Serve: Use an immersion blender to puree the soup until smooth. Adjust the seasoning as needed. Serve hot, garnished with roasted pumpkin seeds for a crunchy texture.

Nutritional Breakdown (Estimated per serving): Calories: 230 kcal, Protein: 2 g, Fat: 7 g (Saturated Fat: 1 g), Carbs: 43 g (Dietary Fiber: 6 g, Sugars: 20 g)

CAULIFLOWER AND TURMERIC SOUP

INGREDIENTS
- 2 tablespoons olive oil
- 1 onion, chopped
- 2 garlic cloves, minced
- 1 butternut squash, peeled, seeded, and cubed
- 2 apples, peeled, cored and chopped
- 4 cups vegetable broth
- 1 teaspoon ground cinnamon
- 1/2 teaspoon ground nutmeg
- Salt and pepper to taste
- Roasted pumpkin seeds for garnish

Preparation time:	Cook time:	Total time:
10 min	25 min	35 min

DIRECTIONS
Cook Onion and Garlic: In a large pot, heat the olive oil over medium heat. Add the onion and garlic, cooking until the onion is soft and translucent.

Add Cauliflower and Turmeric: Mix in the cauliflower and turmeric powder, coating the cauliflower evenly with the turmeric.

Simmer the Soup: Pour the vegetable broth into the pot, seasoning the mixture with salt and pepper to taste. Bring to a boil, reduce the heat, and let it simmer until the cauliflower is tender, about 20 minutes.

Blend and Serve: Puree the soup using an immersion blender until smooth. For a creamier texture, stir in a splash of coconut milk. Serve the soup garnished with fresh parsley.

Nutritional Breakdown (Estimated per serving): Calories: 150 kcal, Protein: 4 g, Fat: 10 g (Saturated Fat: 1.5 g), Carbs: 13 g (Dietary Fiber: 3 g, Sugars: 5 g)

CHAPTER 8: FISH AND SEAFOOD

SALMON AND SPINACH SALAD WITH AVOCADO DRESSING

INGREDIENTS
- 4 salmon fillets (6 oz each)
- 8 cups baby spinach
- 1 avocado, diced
- 1/2 cup cherry tomatoes, halved
- 1/4 cup walnuts, toasted
  For the dressing:
- 1 ripe avocado
- 2 tablespoons lemon juice
- 1 garlic clove, minced
- 1/4 cup olive oil
- Water, as needed, to thin
- Salt and pepper to taste

Preparation time:	Cook time:	Total time:
20 min	15 min	35 min

DIRECTIONS
Cook Salmon: Season salmon with salt and pepper. Cook in a preheated skillet over medium heat for 5-7 minutes per side or until desired doneness.

Prepare Salad: In a large bowl, combine baby spinach, diced avocado, cherry tomatoes, and walnuts.

Blend Dressing: In a blender, combine the avocado, lemon juice, garlic, and olive oil. Blend until smooth, adding water to reach the desired consistency. Season with salt and pepper.

Assemble and Serve: Place cooked salmon on top of the spinach salad. Drizzle with avocado dressing before serving.

Nutritional Breakdown (Estimated per serving): Calories: 450 kcal, Protein: 35 g, Fat: 30 g (Saturated Fat: 5 g), Carbs: 15 g (Dietary Fiber: 7 g, Sugars: 3 g)

GRILLED SHRIMP AND QUINOA SALAD

INGREDIENTS

- 1 lb shrimp, peeled and deveined
- 2 cups cooked quinoa, cooled
- 4 cups arugula
- 1/2 cup diced cucumber
- 1/2 cup cherry tomatoes, halved
    For the dressing:
- 3 tablespoons extra virgin olive oil
- 2 tablespoons orange juice
- 1 tablespoon lime juice
- 1 garlic clove, minced
- Salt and pepper to taste

Preparation time:	Cook time:	Total time:
15 min	10 min	25 min

DIRECTIONS

Grill Shrimp: Season shrimp with salt and pepper. Grill over medium heat for 2-3 minutes per side or until opaque.
Combine Salad: In a large bowl, mix arugula, quinoa, cucumber, and cherry tomatoes.
Prepare Dressing: Whisk together olive oil, orange juice, lime juice, and minced garlic. Season with salt and pepper.
Dress and Serve: Toss the salad with the dressing, top with grilled shrimp, and serve immediately.

Nutritional Breakdown (Estimated per serving): Calories: 380 kcal, Protein: 25 g, Fat: 15 g (Saturated Fat: 2 g), Carbs: 35 g (Dietary Fiber: 5 g, Sugars: 5 g)

BAKED COD WITH MEDITERRANEAN VEGETABLES

INGREDIENTS
- 4 cod fillets (6 oz each)
- 2 cups cherry tomatoes
- 1 zucchini, sliced
- 1 bell pepper, sliced
- 1/4 cup Kalamata olives, pitted
  For the dressing:
- 3 tablespoons olive oil
- 2 tablespoons lemon juice
- 1 teaspoon dried oregano
- 2 garlic cloves, minced
- Salt and pepper to taste

Preparation time:	Cook time:	Total time:
15 min	20 min	35 min

DIRECTIONS
Preheat Oven: Preheat oven to 400°F (200°C). Arrange cod and vegetables on a baking sheet.
Season: Drizzle olive oil and lemon juice over cod and vegetables. Sprinkle with oregano, garlic, salt, and pepper.
Bake: Bake for 20 minutes or until cod is cooked through and vegetables are tender.
Serve: Serve the baked cod with Mediterranean vegetables garnished with Kalamata olives.

Nutritional Breakdown (Estimated per serving): Calories: 300 kcal, Protein: 28 g, Fat: 10 g (Saturated Fat: 1.5 g), Carbs: 25 g (Dietary Fiber: 6 g, Sugars: 8 g)

TUNA AND AVOCADO POKE BOWL

INGREDIENTS
- 2 cups sushi rice, cooked and cooled
- 1 lb sushi-grade tuna, cubed
- 2 avocados, cubed
- 1/2 cup cucumber, thinly sliced
- 1/4 cup scallions, chopped
- 1 tablespoon sesame seeds
    For the dressing:
- 3 tablespoons soy sauce (low sodium, if possible)
- 2 tablespoons sesame oil
- 1 tablespoon rice vinegar
- 1 teaspoon honey (or maple syrup for vegan option)
- Salt and pepper to taste

Preparation time:	Cook time:	Total time:
20 min	0 min	20 min

DIRECTIONS
Prepare Bowls: Divide the sushi rice into 4 bowls. Top with cubed tuna, avocado, cucumber, and scallions.
Mix Dressing: In a small bowl, whisk together soy sauce, sesame oil, rice vinegar, and honey. Season with a pinch of salt and pepper.
Serve: Drizzle the dressing over each bowl, garnish with sesame seeds, and serve immediately.

Nutritional Breakdown (Estimated per serving): Calories: 420 kcal, Protein: 25 g, Fat: 20 g (Saturated Fat: 3 g), Carbs: 35 g (Dietary Fiber: 7 g, Sugars: 5 g)

GARLIC LEMON SCALLOPS WITH ASPARAGUS

INGREDIENTS
- 1 lb scallops
- 2 tablespoons olive oil
- 2 garlic cloves, minced
- 1 lemon, juiced and zested
- 2 cups asparagus, trimmed
- Salt and pepper to taste

Preparation time:	Cook time:	Total time:
10 min	10 min	20 min

DIRECTIONS
Cook Scallops: Heat olive oil in a large skillet over medium-high heat. Season scallops with salt and pepper, add to the skillet, and cook until golden brown on each side, about 2-3 minutes per side.

Sauté Asparagus: In the same skillet, add a bit more oil if needed, then add garlic and asparagus. Cook until asparagus is tender-crisp, about 5 minutes. Stir in lemon juice and zest.

Serve: Arrange scallops over asparagus and serve immediately. This dish features the anti-inflammatory power of garlic and lemon, paired with the lean protein of scallops.

Nutritional Breakdown (Estimated per serving): Calories: 250 kcal, Protein: 20 g, Fat: 12 g (Saturated Fat: 2 g), Carbs: 15 g (Dietary Fiber: 3 g, Sugars: 2 g)

GRILLED MACKEREL WITH HERB SALAD

INGREDIENTS
- 4 mackerel fillets
- 2 tablespoons olive oil
- Salt and pepper to taste
- 4 cups mixed herbs (parsley, cilantro, dill), roughly chopped
- 1 lemon, for serving

Preparation time:	Cook time:	Total time:
15 min	10 min	25 min

DIRECTIONS
Grill Mackerel: Preheat the grill to medium-high heat. Brush mackerel fillets with olive oil and season with salt and pepper. Grill for 5 minutes per side or until cooked through.

Prepare Herb Salad: In a bowl, combine the chopped herbs. Dress lightly with olive oil, salt, and pepper.

Serve: Place grilled mackerel on plates, accompanied by the fresh herb salad. Serve with lemon wedges on the side.

Nutritional Breakdown (Estimated per serving): Calories: 310 kcal, Protein: 23 g, Fat: 22 g (Saturated Fat: 5 g), Carbs: 3 g (Dietary Fiber: 1 g, Sugars: 1 g)

BAKED HADDOCK WITH TOMATO AND OLIVES

INGREDIENTS
- 4 haddock fillets (6 oz each)
- 2 tablespoons olive oil
- 1 cup cherry tomatoes, halved
- 1/2 cup Kalamata olives, pitted and halved
- 1/4 cup fresh basil leaves, chopped
- 2 garlic cloves, minced
- Salt and pepper to taste

Preparation time:	Cook time:	Total time:
10 min	20 min	30 min

DIRECTIONS

Preheat Oven: Preheat your oven to 375°F (190°C). Arrange haddock fillets in a baking dish.

Season and Add Toppings: Drizzle fillets with olive oil and season with salt and pepper. Scatter cherry tomatoes, Kalamata olives, and minced garlic over and around the fish.

Bake: Place in the oven and bake for 15-20 minutes or until the fish flakes easily with a fork.

Garnish and Serve: Just before serving, sprinkle fresh basil over the baked haddock. This Mediterranean-inspired dish is not only flavorful but also packed with anti-inflammatory ingredients like tomatoes, olives, and garlic.

Nutritional Breakdown (Estimated per serving): Calories: 210 kcal, Protein: 27 g, Fat: 8 g (Saturated Fat: 1 g), Carbs: 8 g (Dietary Fiber: 2 g, Sugars: 4 g)

CHILI LIME SHRIMP TACOS

INGREDIENTS
- 1 lb shrimp, peeled and deveined
- 1 tablespoon olive oil
- 1 teaspoon chili powder
- Juice and zest of 1 lime
- Salt and pepper to taste
- 8 small corn tortillas, warmed
- 2 cups cabbage, shredded
- 1 avocado, sliced
- 1/4 cup cilantro, chopped
- Lime wedges for serving

Preparation time:	Cook time:	Total time:
20 min	10 min	30 min

DIRECTIONS
Marinate Shrimp: In a bowl, combine shrimp with olive oil, chili powder, lime juice, and zest. Season with salt and pepper. Let marinate for 10-15 minutes.
Cook Shrimp: Heat a large skillet over medium-high heat. Add shrimp and cook for 2-3 minutes per side or until pink and cooked through.
Assemble Tacos: Fill each tortilla with a handful of shredded cabbage, a few shrimp, slices of avocado, and a sprinkle of cilantro.
Serve: Offer lime wedges on the side for squeezing over tacos.

Nutritional Breakdown (Estimated per serving): Calories: 210 kcal, Protein: 27 g, Fat: 8 g (Saturated Fat: 1 g), Carbs: 8 g (Dietary Fiber: 2 g, Sugars: 4 g)

CHAPTER 9: POULTRY

GINGER HONEY GLAZED CHICKEN THIGHS

INGREDIENTS
- 8 chicken thighs, skin on
- 2 tablespoons grated ginger
- 1/4 cup honey
- 2 tablespoons soy sauce
- 1 tablespoon olive oil
- Salt and pepper to taste
- Sesame seeds and green onions for garnish

Preparation time:	Cook time:	Total time:
15 min	25 min	40 min

DIRECTIONS
Preheat Oven: Preheat your oven to 375°F (190°C).
Prepare Glaze: Mix ginger, honey, and soy sauce in a bowl.
Cook Chicken: Season chicken thighs with salt and pepper. In a skillet, sear them skin-side down in olive oil until golden. Flip, then brush with the glaze.
Bake: Transfer to the oven and bake for 20 minutes, glazing occasionally.
Garnish and Serve: Sprinkle with sesame seeds and chopped green onions before serving.

Nutritional Breakdown (Estimated per serving): Calories: 400 kcal, Protein: 30 g, Fat: 22 g (Saturated Fat: 5 g), Carbs: 20 g (Dietary Fiber: 0 g, Sugars: 18 g)

LEMON AND ROSEMARY CHICKEN BREAST

INGREDIENTS
- 4 boneless, skinless chicken breasts
- 2 tablespoons olive oil
- Juice and zest of 1 lemon
- 2 tablespoons fresh rosemary, chopped
- Salt and pepper to taste

Preparation time:	Cook time:	Total time:
10 min	20 min	30 min

DIRECTIONS
Marinate Chicken: Combine lemon juice, zest, rosemary, salt, and pepper. Marinate the chicken in this mixture for at least 30 minutes.

Cook Chicken: In a skillet over medium heat, cook the chicken in olive oil until golden on each side and cooked through, about 10 minutes per side.

Serve: Drizzle any remaining pan juices over the chicken before serving.

Nutritional Breakdown (Estimated per serving): Calories: 310 kcal, Protein: 26 g, Fat: 18 g (Saturated Fat: 3 g), Carbs: 5 g (Dietary Fiber: 1 g, Sugars: 1 g)

SPICY CHICKEN AND VEGGIE STIR-FRY

INGREDIENTS

- 2 tablespoons coconut oil
- 1 lb chicken breast, thinly sliced
- 2 cups broccoli florets
- 1 bell pepper, sliced
- 1 carrot, julienned
- 2 teaspoons ginger, minced
- 2 garlic cloves, minced
    For the sauce:
- 2 tablespoons soy sauce (low sodium)
- 1 tablespoon honey
- 1 tablespoon apple cider vinegar
- 1 teaspoon chili flakes (adjust to taste)
- Salt and pepper to taste

Preparation time:	Cook time:	Total time:
15 min	15 min	30 min

DIRECTIONS

Prepare Sauce: Whisk together soy sauce, honey, apple cider vinegar, and chili flakes in a small bowl. Set aside.

Cook Chicken: Heat coconut oil in a large skillet or wok over medium-high heat. Add chicken slices and cook until browned and cooked through. Remove chicken and set aside.

Stir-Fry Veggies: In the same skillet, add a bit more oil if needed. Stir-fry broccoli, bell pepper, carrot, ginger, and garlic until the vegetables are tender.

Combine: Return the chicken to the skillet. Pour the sauce over the chicken and vegetables. Stir well to combine and cook for another 2-3 minutes.

Serve: Serve hot. This dish combines ginger and garlic's anti-inflammatory benefits with chicken's lean protein and the nutrient density of colorful vegetables.

Nutritional Breakdown (Estimated per serving): Calories: 280 kcal, Protein: 26 g, Fat: 9 g (Saturated Fat: 1.5 g), Carbs: 22 g (Dietary Fiber: 5 g, Sugars: 8 g)

HONEY MUSTARD CHICKEN WITH ROASTED BRUSSELS SPROUTS

INGREDIENTS

- 4 boneless, skinless chicken breasts
- 2 tablespoons Dijon mustard
- 2 tablespoons honey
- 1 tablespoon olive oil
- 1 teaspoon apple cider vinegar
- Salt and pepper to taste
- 2 cups Brussels sprouts, halved
- 1 tablespoon olive oil
- Salt and pepper to taste

Preparation time:	Cook time:	Total time:
15 min	25 min	40 min

DIRECTIONS

Preheat Oven: Preheat your oven to 400°F (200°C). Line a baking sheet with parchment paper.

Prepare Chicken: In a small bowl, whisk together Dijon mustard, honey, 1 tablespoon of olive oil, and apple cider vinegar. Season the mixture with salt and pepper.

Marinate: Place chicken breasts in a large bowl. Pour the honey mustard mixture over the chicken, ensuring each piece is well-coated. Let marinate for at least 10 minutes.

Prepare Brussels Sprouts: Toss halved Brussels sprouts with 1 tablespoon olive oil, salt, and pepper.

Cook: Arrange chicken breasts and Brussels sprouts on the prepared baking sheet. Bake for 25 minutes, or until the chicken is cooked through and Brussels sprouts are caramelized.

Serve: Serve the honey mustard chicken with roasted Brussels sprouts on the side. This meal combines the tangy sweetness of honey mustard with the earthy, rich flavor of roasted Brussels sprouts, offering a delightful balance of taste and nutritional benefits.

Nutritional Breakdown (Estimated per serving): Calories: 310 kcal, Protein: 27 g, Fat: 12 g (Saturated Fat: 2 g), Carbs: 25 g (Dietary Fiber: 6 g, Sugars: 12 g)

CHAPTER 10: SIDE DISHES AND SNACKS

AVOCADO HUMMUS

INGREDIENTS
- 1 ripe avocado
- 1 can (15 ounces) chickpeas, drained and rinsed
- 2 tablespoons tahini
- Juice of 1 lemon
- 1 garlic clove, minced
- Salt and pepper to taste
- 2 tablespoons olive oil
- Paprika for garnish

Preparation time:	Cook time:	Total time:
10 min	0 min	10 min

DIRECTIONS
Blend Ingredients: In a food processor, combine avocado, chickpeas, tahini, lemon juice, and garlic. Season with salt and pepper.
Process Until Smooth: Blend until creamy, gradually adding olive oil until the desired consistency is reached.
Serve: Garnish with paprika. Serve with vegetable sticks or gluten-free pita chips for dipping.

Nutritional Breakdown (Estimated per serving): Calories: 150 kcal, Protein: 4 g, Fat: 12 g (Saturated Fat: 2 g), Carbs: 9 g (Dietary Fiber: 5 g, Sugars: 1 g)

ROASTED SPICED CAULIFLOWER

INGREDIENTS

- 1 head cauliflower, cut into florets
- 2 tablespoons olive oil
- 1 teaspoon turmeric
- 1 teaspoon cumin
- Salt and pepper to taste

Preparation time:	Cook time:	Total time:
10 min	25 min	35 min

DIRECTIONS

Preheat Oven: Preheat your oven to 425°F (220°C).
Season Cauliflower: Toss cauliflower florets with olive oil, turmeric, cumin, salt, and pepper.
Roast: Spread the florets on a baking sheet and roast for 25 minutes or until golden and tender.
Serve: Enjoy as a flavorful and anti-inflammatory side dish.

Nutritional Breakdown (Estimated per serving): Calories: 120 kcal, Protein: 4 g, Fat: 7 g (Saturated Fat: 1 g), Carbs: 12 g (Dietary Fiber: 5 g, Sugars: 4 g)

ZESTY LIME AND CILANTRO QUINOA

INGREDIENTS

- 1 cup quinoa, rinsed
- 2 cups water
- Juice and zest of 2 limes
- 1/4 cup cilantro, chopped
- 1 garlic clove, minced
- Salt and pepper to taste
- 2 tablespoons olive oil

Preparation time:	Cook time:	Total time:
10 min	15 min	25 min

DIRECTIONS

Cook Quinoa: In a saucepan, bring quinoa and water to a boil. Reduce heat, cover, and simmer for 15 minutes or until water is absorbed.

Flavor: Fluff quinoa with a fork and transfer to a bowl. While still warm, add lime juice, zest, cilantro, and minced garlic. Season with salt and pepper.

Finish: Drizzle with olive oil and toss until everything is evenly mixed.

Serve: This can be enjoyed warm or cold as a flavorful, nutrient-rich side dish.

Nutritional Breakdown (Estimated per serving): Calories: 220 kcal, Protein: 8 g, Fat: 5 g (Saturated Fat: 0.5 g), Carbs: 35 g (Dietary Fiber: 5 g, Sugars: 1 g)

GARLIC ROASTED BRUSSELS SPROUTS

INGREDIENTS
- 1 lb Brussels sprouts, halved
- 3 tablespoons olive oil
- 4 garlic cloves, minced
- Salt and pepper to taste

Preparation time:	Cook time:	Total time:
10 min	20 min	30 min

DIRECTIONS
Prep: Preheat oven to 400°F (200°C). Toss Brussels sprouts with olive oil and garlic in a bowl. Season with salt and pepper.
Roast: Spread on a baking sheet in a single layer. Roast for 20 minutes until crispy on the outside and tender on the inside.
Serve: Adjust seasoning if necessary and serve hot.

Nutritional Breakdown (Estimated per serving): Calories: 120 kcal, Protein: 4 g, Fat: 7 g (Saturated Fat: 1 g), Carbs: 12 g (Dietary Fiber: 4 g, Sugars: 3 g)

SPICY SWEET POTATO WEDGES

INGREDIENTS
- 2 large sweet potatoes, cut into wedges
- 2 tablespoons olive oil
- 1 teaspoon smoked paprika
- 1/2 teaspoon cayenne pepper
- Salt and pepper to taste

Preparation time:	Cook time:	Total time:
10 min	30 min	40 min

DIRECTIONS
Season: In a large bowl, toss sweet potato wedges with olive oil, smoked paprika, cayenne pepper, salt, and pepper.
Bake: Arrange on a baking sheet and bake at 425°F (220°C) for 30 minutes, flipping halfway through, until edges are crispy.
Enjoy: Serve warm as a flavorful snack or side, perfect for dipping in your favorite sauce.

Nutritional Breakdown (Estimated per serving): Calories: 200 kcal, Protein: 2 g, Fat: 9 g (Saturated Fat: 1.3 g), Carbs: 28 g (Dietary Fiber: 4 g, Sugars: 6 g)

GRILLED ASPARAGUS WITH LEMON ZEST

INGREDIENTS
- 1 lb asparagus, trimmed
- 2 tablespoons olive oil
- Zest of 1 lemon
- Salt and pepper to taste

Preparation time:	Cook time:	Total time:
10 min	10 min	20 min

DIRECTIONS
Prep Asparagus: Toss the asparagus with olive oil, lemon zest, salt, and pepper.

Grill: Heat a grill or grill pan over medium-high heat. Grill the asparagus on each side for 3-5 minutes or until tender and charred.

Serve: Plate the grilled asparagus, adding a final sprinkle of lemon zest and sea salt before serving. This side dish offers a delightful blend of smoky flavors with a hint of citrus, making it a perfect complement to any main course.

Nutritional Breakdown (Estimated per serving): Calories: 75 kcal, Protein: 3 g, Fat: 5 g (Saturated Fat: 0.7 g), Carbs: 6 g (Dietary Fiber: 3 g, Sugars: 3 g)

ROASTED CHICKPEAS WITH ROSEMARY AND SEA SALT

INGREDIENTS
- 1 can (15 ounces) of chickpeas, drained, rinsed, and dried
- 2 tablespoons olive oil
- 1 tablespoon fresh rosemary, chopped
- 1/2 teaspoon sea salt
- 1/4 teaspoon cracked black pepper

Preparation time:	Cook time:	Total time:
5 min	40 min	45 min

DIRECTIONS
Preheat Oven: Preheat your oven to 375°F (190°C).
Season: In a bowl, toss the chickpeas with olive oil, chopped rosemary, sea salt, and pepper until evenly coated.
Roast: Spread the chickpeas in a single layer on a baking sheet. Roast for 35-40 minutes, stirring occasionally, until crispy and golden.
Enjoy: Serve these crunchy chickpeas as a healthy, savory snack or a garnish for salads and soups.

Nutritional Breakdown (Estimated per serving): Calories: 150 kcal, Protein: 5 g, Fat: 7 g (Saturated Fat: 1 g), Carbs: 18 g (Dietary Fiber: 5 g, Sugars: 3 g)

SWEET POTATO CHIPS WITH CINNAMON AND PAPRIKA

INGREDIENTS
- 2 large sweet potatoes, thinly sliced
- 1 tablespoon olive oil
- 1/2 teaspoon ground cinnamon
- 1/2 teaspoon paprika
- Salt to taste

Preparation time:	Cook time:	Total time:
15 min	20 min	35 min

DIRECTIONS
Preheat Oven: Preheat your oven to 400°F (200°C). Line two baking sheets with parchment paper for easy cleanup.

Prepare Sweet Potatoes: Use a mandoline or sharp knife to slice the sweet potatoes into thin, even chips.

Season: In a large bowl, toss the sweet potato slices with olive oil, cinnamon, paprika, and a pinch of salt, ensuring each slice is evenly coated.

Arrange: Spread the sweet potato slices in a single layer on the prepared baking sheets, ensuring they don't overlap to ensure even cooking.

Bake: Bake in the preheated oven for 10 minutes, flip the chips, and continue baking for another 8-10 minutes or until crispy and slightly browned at the edges. Watch them closely towards the end to prevent burning.

Cool and Serve: Let the chips cool on the baking sheet for a few minutes; they will continue to crisp up as they cool. Serve as a healthy, crunchy snack or side dish.

Nutritional Breakdown (Estimated per serving): Calories: 120 kcal, Protein: 1 g, Fat: 4 g (Saturated Fat: 0.5 g), Carbs: 20 g (Dietary Fiber: 3 g, Sugars: 4 g)

CHAPTER 11: DESSERTS

VEGAN APPLE TART WITH WALNUT CRUST

INGREDIENTS
For the Walnut Crust:

- 1 1/2 cups walnuts
- 1 cup rolled oats
- 1/4 cup ground flaxseed
- 1/4 cup coconut oil, melted
- 2 tablespoons maple syrup
- A pinch of salt

For the Apple Filling:

- 3 large apples, peeled, cored, and thinly sliced
- 2 tablespoons maple syrup
- 1 teaspoon cinnamon
- 1/2 teaspoon nutmeg
- 1 tablespoon lemon juice

For the Glaze:

- 1 tablespoon apricot jam or preserve
- 1 tablespoon water

Nutritional Breakdown (Estimated per serving):
Calories: 250 kcal, Protein: 4 g, Fat: 15 g (Saturated Fat: 2 g), Carbs: 28 g (Dietary Fiber: 4 g, Sugars: 12 g)

Preparation time:	Cook time:	Total time:
20 min	35 min	55 min

DIRECTIONS
Preheat Oven: Preheat your oven to 350°F (175°C). Lightly grease a 9-inch tart pan with a removable bottom.
Make the Crust: In a food processor, combine the walnuts, rolled oats, ground flaxseed, melted coconut oil, maple syrup, and a pinch of salt. Process until the mixture comes together and forms a sticky dough. Press the dough evenly into the bottom and up the sides of the prepared tart pan.
Pre-bake the Crust: Bake the crust in the preheated oven for 10-12 minutes or until it begins to turn golden. Remove from the oven and let cool slightly.
Prepare the Apple Filling: In a large bowl, toss the thinly sliced apples with maple syrup, cinnamon, nutmeg, and lemon juice until well coated.
Arrange the Apples: Arrange the apple slices in the pre-baked crust, slightly overlapping each other in a circular pattern starting from the outer edge and working your way to the center.
Bake: Bake the tart in the oven for about 20-25 minutes, or until the apples are tender and the crust is a deep golden brown.
Glaze the Tart: Heat the apricot jam with water in a small saucepan over low heat until melted and smooth. Brush the glaze over the warm tart to give it a shiny finish.
Cool and Serve: Allow the tart to cool in the pan on a wire rack. Once cooled, remove the tart from the pan, slice, and serve.

GINGER SPICED COOKIES

INGREDIENTS
- 1 1/4 cups almond flour
- 1/4 cup coconut flour
- 1 tsp baking powder
- 1/4 tsp salt
- 2 tsp ground ginger
- 1 tsp cinnamon
- 1/4 tsp ground cloves
- 1/4 tsp ground turmeric
- 1/4 cup coconut oil, melted
- 1/2 cup maple syrup
- 1 tsp vanilla extract
- 1 tbsp fresh ginger, grated

Nutritional Breakdown (Estimated per serving, per cookie): Calories: 90 kcal, Protein: 2 g, Fat: 4 g (Saturated Fat: 0.5 g), Carbs: 12 g (Dietary Fiber: 1 g, Sugars: 6 g)

Preparation time:	Cook time:	Total time:
15 min	10 min	25 min

DIRECTIONS

Dry Ingredients: In a large mixing bowl, whisk together almond flour, coconut flour, baking powder, salt, ground ginger, cinnamon, cloves, and turmeric. These spices not only add flavor but also offer anti-inflammatory benefits.

Wet Ingredients: In a separate bowl, mix the melted coconut oil, maple syrup, vanilla extract, and grated fresh ginger. Fresh ginger is a potent anti-inflammatory agent and adds a vibrant kick to the cookies.

Combine: Pour the wet ingredients into the dry ingredients and stir until a dough forms. If the dough is too sticky, add a bit more almond flour until it's manageable.

Chill the Dough: Wrap the dough in plastic wrap and chill in the refrigerator for at least 30 minutes. This helps the flavors to meld and makes the dough easier to handle.

Preheat Oven: Preheat your oven to 350°F (175°C) and line a baking sheet with parchment paper.

Form Cookies: Once chilled, roll the dough into balls (about 1 tablespoon per cookie) and place them on the prepared baking sheet. Flatten each ball slightly with your fingers or the bottom of a glass.

Bake: Bake for 10-12 minutes or until the edges turn golden brown. The cookies will still be soft but will firm up as they cool.

Cool: Allow the cookies to cool on the baking sheet for 5 minutes before transferring them to a wire rack to cool completely.

PEACH GALETTE

INGREDIENTS

For the Crust:
- 1 1/2 cups gluten-free all-purpose flour
- 1/4 cup cold unsalted butter or coconut oil, cubed
- 1/4 teaspoon salt
- 4-6 tablespoons ice-cold water
- 1 teaspoon apple cider vinegar

For the Filling:
- 4 medium peaches, pitted and sliced
- 2 tablespoons maple syrup or honey
- 1 teaspoon ground cinnamon
- 1/2 teaspoon ground ginger
- 1/4 teaspoon ground turmeric
- 2 teaspoons lemon juice
- 1 tablespoon cornstarch or tapioca flour (for thickening)

For the Glaze (Optional):
- 1 tablespoon apricot jam
- 1 tablespoon water

Nutritional Breakdown (Estimated per serving):
Calories: 190 kcal, Protein: 3 g, Fat: 9 g (Saturated Fat: 1.5 g), Carbs: 27 g (Dietary Fiber: 3 g, Sugars: 12 g)

Preparation time:	Cook time:	Total time:
20 min	25 min	45 min

DIRECTIONS

Prepare the Dough: In a large mixing bowl, whisk together the gluten-free flour and salt. Add the cold butter or coconut oil and use a pastry cutter or your fingers to work it into the flour until the mixture resembles coarse crumbs.

Mix in the apple cider vinegar. Gradually add ice-cold water, 1 tablespoon at a time, mixing until the dough comes together in a ball. You may not need all the water.

Flatten the dough into a disk, wrap it in plastic wrap, and chill in the refrigerator for at least 30 minutes.

Prepare the Filling: In a large bowl, combine the sliced peaches, maple syrup (or honey), cinnamon, ginger, turmeric, lemon juice, and corn-starch. Toss gently to coat the peaches evenly.

Preheat the Oven: Preheat your oven to 375°F (190°C). Line a baking sheet with parchment paper.

Assemble the Galette: On a lightly floured surface, roll out the chilled dough into a 12-inch circle. Transfer to the prepared baking sheet.

Arrange the peach filling in the center of the dough, leaving a 2-inch border. Fold the edges of the dough over the peaches, pleating as necessary to hold the filling in.

Bake: Bake for 25-30 minutes, or until the crust is golden brown and the filling is bubbly.

Prepare the Glaze (Optional): While the galette bakes, warm the apricot jam and water in a small saucepan over low heat until the jam melts. Strain if necessary to remove any fruit pieces. Brush the glaze over the hot galette when it comes out of the oven for a glossy finish.

Cool and Serve: Allow the galette to cool for a few minutes before cutting into slices. Serve warm or at room temperature for a delicious and healthful dessert.

CHERRY SORBET

INGREDIENTS

- 4 cups fresh or frozen cherries, pitted
- 1/2 cup water
- 1/3 cup honey or maple syrup (adjust to taste)
- 2 tablespoons lemon juice
- 1 teaspoon grated ginger
- 1/2 teaspoon ground turmeric

Preparation time:	Cook time:	Total time:
10 min	5 min	15 min

DIRECTIONS

Prepare the Cherry Mixture: If using fresh cherries, pit them first. Combine the cherries, water, honey (or maple syrup), lemon juice, grated ginger, and ground turmeric in a medium saucepan. Bring the mixture to a simmer over medium heat, stirring occasionally. Allow to simmer for about 5 minutes or until the cherries are soft and the flavors have melded together. The ginger and turmeric add a potent anti-inflammatory boost to the sorbet.

Cool and Blend: Remove the cherry mixture from the heat and let it cool to room temperature. Once cooled, transfer the mixture to a blender or food processor.

Blend until smooth. If you prefer a sorbet without cherry bits, you can strain the mixture through a fine mesh sieve to achieve a smoother consistency.

Freeze: Pour the blended cherry mixture into a shallow baking dish or a sorbet machine if you have one. If using a baking dish, place it in the freezer.

For the first hour, stir the mixture every 15 minutes to break up any ice crystals, ensuring a smoother texture. Continue freezing until the sorbet is firm, typically around 3-4 hours.

Serve: Before serving, let the sorbet sit at room temperature for a few minutes to soften slightly for easier scooping. Serve in bowls or glasses, garnished with a sprig of mint or a few fresh cherries for an elegant presentation.

Nutritional Breakdown (Estimated per serving):
Calories: 130 kcal, Protein: 2 g, Fat: 0 g, Carbs: 33 g (Dietary Fiber: 2 g, Sugars: 28 g)

BANANA NUT OATMEAL CUPS

INGREDIENTS
- 3 ripe bananas, mashed
- 2 cups old-fashioned oats (gluten-free if necessary)
- 1/4 cup walnuts, chopped (plus extra for topping)
- 1/4 cup almonds, chopped
- 1/4 cup hemp seeds
- 2 tablespoons flaxseed meal
- 1 teaspoon cinnamon
- 1/2 teaspoon ground turmeric
- 1/4 teaspoon ground ginger
- 1 teaspoon baking powder
- 1/4 teaspoon salt
- 1 cup almond milk
- 1/4 cup maple syrup
- 1 teaspoon vanilla extract

Nutritional Breakdown (Estimated per serving, 1 cup): Calories: 150 kcal, Protein: 4 g, Fat: 7 g (Saturated Fat: 1 g), Carbs: 20 g (Dietary Fiber: 3 g, Sugars: 7 g)

Preparation time:	Cook time:	Total time:
10 min	20 min	30 min

DIRECTIONS

Preheat the Oven: Preheat your oven to 350°F (175°C). Prepare a 12-cup muffin tin by greasing it with coconut oil or lining it with paper liners.

Combine Dry Ingredients: In a large mixing bowl, combine the oats, chopped walnuts, almonds, hemp seeds, flaxseed meal, cinnamon, turmeric, ginger, baking powder, and salt. Mix well to distribute the spices evenly.

Add Wet Ingredients: To the same bowl, add the mashed bananas, almond milk, maple syrup, and vanilla extract. Stir until all the ingredients are well combined and moistened throughout the mixture.

Fill Muffin Cups: Spoon the oatmeal mixture evenly into the prepared muffin cups, filling each nearly to the top. Sprinkle additional chopped walnuts over each cup, if desired, for extra crunch and flavor.

Bake: Place the muffin tin in the oven and bake for 20-25 minutes, or until the tops of the oatmeal cups are set and lightly golden.

Cool and Serve: Allow the oatmeal cups to cool in the pan for 5 minutes, then transfer them to a wire rack to cool completely. These cups are delicious and served warm or at room temperature.

Storage: Store any leftover oatmeal cups in an airtight container in the refrigerator for up to 5 days. They can also be frozen for up to 3 months. Warm briefly in the microwave before serving for a quick and nutritious breakfast or snack.

RASPBERRY COBBLER

INGREDIENTS

For the Filling:
- 4 cups fresh or frozen raspberries
- 1/4 cup honey or pure maple syrup
- 1 tablespoon chia seeds (for thickening and adding omega-3 fatty acids)
- 1 teaspoon vanilla extract
- 1 teaspoon lemon zest
- 1 tablespoon lemon juice
- 1/2 teaspoon ground cinnamon
- 1/4 teaspoon ground ginger

For the Topping:
- 1 cup gluten-free all-purpose flour (ensure it includes xanthan gum if your blend doesn't)
- 1/4 cup almond meal
- 2 tablespoons coconut sugar (or substitute with brown sugar)
- 1 teaspoon baking powder
- 1/4 teaspoon salt
- 1/4 cup cold unsalted butter or coconut oil
- 1/2 cup almond milk

Preparation time:	Cook time:	Total time:
15 min	30 min	45 min

DIRECTIONS

Preheat the Oven: Preheat your oven to 375°F (190°C). Grease an 8-inch square baking dish or a similar-sized round pie dish.

Prepare the Filling: In a large bowl, mix the raspberries, honey (or maple syrup), chia seeds, vanilla extract, lemon zest, lemon juice, cinnamon, and ginger until well combined. Pour the raspberry mixture into the prepared baking dish, spreading it out evenly.

Make the Topping: In a medium bowl, whisk together the gluten-free flour, almond meal, coconut sugar, baking powder, and salt. Cut in the cold butter or coconut oil using a pastry blender or two knives until the mixture resembles coarse crumbs. Stir in the almond milk until the dough comes together; do not overmix.

Assemble the Cobbler: Drop spoonfuls of the topping over the raspberry filling, covering it as much as possible. It's okay if some of the filling peeks through; this will add to the rustic charm of the cobbler.

Bake: Bake in the preheated oven for 30-35 minutes or until the topping is golden brown and the raspberry filling is bubbling around the edges.

Cool and Serve: Let the cobbler cool for 10 minutes before serving. This dessert is delicious on its own or served with a dollop of whipped coconut cream or vanilla ice cream for an extra special treat.

Nutritional Breakdown (Estimated per serving): Calories: 220 kcal, Protein: 3 g, Fat: 8 g (Saturated Fat: 5 g), Carbs: 36 g (Dietary Fiber: 5 g, Sugars: 15 g)

CHAPTER 12: SMOOTHIES AND DRINKS

STRAWBERRY BANANA SMOOTHIE

INGREDIENTS
- 1 cup unsweetened almond milk
- 1 ripe banana, sliced
- 1 cup fresh or frozen strawberries
- 1/2 teaspoon ground turmeric (for anti-inflammatory properties)
- 1/2 teaspoon ground ginger (for digestion and inflammation)
- 1 tablespoon ground flaxseeds or chia seeds (for omega-3 fatty acids and fiber)
- 1 teaspoon honey or pure maple syrup (optional for sweetness)
- A pinch of black pepper (to enhance absorption of turmeric)
- Ice cubes (optional for a colder smoothie)

Preparation time:	Cook time:	Total time:
5 min	0 min	5 min

DIRECTIONS
Blend Ingredients: In a blender, add the almond milk, banana, strawberries, turmeric, ginger, flaxseeds or chia seeds, and honey or maple syrup if desired. Don't forget the pinch of black pepper to boost the bioavailability of curcumin in turmeric.

Process Until Smooth: Blend on high speed until the mixture becomes creamy and smooth. If the smoothie seems too thick, add more almond milk to adjust the consistency. For a cooler beverage, add ice cubes to the mix before blending.

Serve Immediately: Pour the smoothie into serving glasses. You can garnish with a few slices of strawberry or a sprinkle of turmeric on top for a decorative touch.

Enjoy: Savor this strawberry banana smoothie as a nutritious breakfast or a refreshing snack. Its anti-inflammatory ingredients make it an excellent choice for supporting overall health and well-being.

Nutritional Breakdown (Estimated per serving): Calories: 180 kcal, Protein: 3 g, Fat: 1 g (Saturated Fat: 0 g), Carbs: 42 g (Dietary Fiber: 5 g, Sugars: 27 g)

RASPBERRY MANGO PEACH SMOOTHIE

INGREDIENTS

- 1 cup coconut water
- 1 cup fresh or frozen raspberries
- 1 ripe mango, peeled and cubed
- 1 ripe peach, sliced (or 1 cup frozen peach slices)
- 1 tablespoon ground flaxseed or chia seeds (for omega-3 fatty acids and fiber)
- 1/2 teaspoon ground turmeric (for anti-inflammatory properties)
- 1/4 teaspoon ground ginger (for digestion and inflammation)
- Ice cubes (optional for a chilled smoothie)

Preparation time:	Cook time:	Total time:
5 min	0 min	5 min

DIRECTIONS

Blend Ingredients: In a blender, combine the coconut water, raspberries, mango, peach, flaxseed or chia seeds, turmeric, and ginger. Add a few ice cubes to the blender if you prefer a colder smoothie.

Process Until Smooth: Blend everything on high until you achieve a smooth and creamy consistency. If the smoothie is too thick, add more coconut water to adjust it to your liking.

Serve Immediately: Once the smoothie reaches your desired consistency, pour it into glasses. You can garnish with a few raspberries or a slice of peach on the rim of the glass for an extra touch of flavor and presentation.

Enjoy: This raspberry mango peach smoothie is delicious and packed with anti-inflammatory ingredients. It's perfect for a refreshing start to your day or as a nutritious snack to help reduce inflammation and support your overall health.

Nutritional Breakdown (Estimated per serving): Calories: 200 kcal, Protein: 3 g, Fat: 1 g (Saturated Fat: 0 g), Carbs: 48 g (Dietary Fiber: 6 g, Sugars: 40 g)

PINEAPPLE AND TURMERIC SMOOTHIE

INGREDIENTS
- 1 cup coconut water or unsweetened almond milk
- 1 cup pineapple chunks (fresh or frozen)
- 1 ripe banana, sliced
- 1/2 teaspoon ground turmeric
- 1/2 inch fresh ginger, peeled and grated
- 1 tablespoon chia seeds or flaxseed meal (for omega-3 fatty acids and fiber)
- Juice of 1/2 lime
- A pinch of black pepper (to enhance the absorption of turmeric)
- Ice cubes (optional for a chilled smoothie)

Preparation time:	Cook time:	Total time:
5 min	0 min	5 min

DIRECTIONS

Blend Ingredients: In a blender, combine the coconut water or almond milk, pineapple chunks, banana, turmeric, ginger, chia seeds or flaxseed meal, lime juice, and a pinch of black pepper. If you prefer a colder smoothie, add ice cubes to the mixture.

Process Until Smooth: Blend on high speed until all ingredients are thoroughly mixed and the smoothie has a creamy consistency. If the smoothie seems too thick, you can adjust its thickness by adding a little more coconut water or almond milk.

Serve Immediately: Once your smoothie is ready, pour it into glasses. You can garnish with a slice of pineapple or a sprinkle of turmeric on top for a visually appealing presentation.

Nutritional Breakdown (Estimated per serving): Calories: 180 kcal, Protein: 2 g, Fat: 1 g (Saturated Fat: 0 g), Carbs: 44 g (Dietary Fiber: 5 g, Sugars: 33 g)

TURMERIC GINGER SMOOTHIE

INGREDIENTS

- 1 cup almond milk
- 1 banana
- 1/2 cup frozen mango chunks
- 1/2 teaspoon turmeric
- 1/2 teaspoon grated ginger
- 1 tablespoon chia seeds
- 1 teaspoon lemon juice
- A pinch of black pepper

Preparation time:	Cook time:	Total time:
5 min	0 min	5 min

DIRECTIONS

Blend Ingredients: In a blender, combine almond milk, banana, mango chunks, turmeric, ginger, chia seeds, lemon juice, and black pepper. Blend until smooth.
Serve: Pour into glasses and serve immediately for a refreshing, anti-inflammatory boost.

Nutritional Breakdown (Estimated per serving): Calories: 180 kcal, Protein: 4 g, Fat: 3 g (Saturated Fat: 0.5 g), Carbs: 36 g (Dietary Fiber: 5 g, Sugars: 25 g)

GINGER LEMON HONEY TEA

INGREDIENTS
- 2 cups water
- 1-inch piece of fresh ginger root peeled and thinly sliced
- Juice of 1/2 lemon
- 2 tablespoons honey, or to taste

Preparation time:	Cook time:	Total time:
5 min	10 min	15 min

DIRECTIONS

Boil Ginger: In a small saucepan, bring the water to a boil. Add the sliced ginger and reduce the heat to simmer. Allow the ginger to steep in the boiling water for about 10 minutes. The longer it simmers, the stronger the ginger flavor will be.

Add Lemon and Honey: Remove the saucepan from the heat. Stir in the lemon juice and honey, adjusting the amounts to suit your taste. Stir until the honey is completely dissolved.

Serve: Strain the tea into mugs to remove the ginger slices. If desired, add a slice of lemon to each mug for decoration and extra lemon flavor.

GOLDEN TURMERIC TEA RECIPE

INGREDIENTS

- 2 cups water or unsweetened almond milk (for a creamier version)
- 1 tablespoon fresh turmeric root, grated (or 1 teaspoon turmeric powder)
- 1 tablespoon fresh ginger root, grated
- 1/4 teaspoon black pepper
- 1 cinnamon stick (or 1/2 teaspoon ground cinnamon)
- 1 tablespoon honey or pure maple syrup (optional for sweetness)
- 1 tablespoon virgin coconut oil (optional, for healthy fats and to further boost absorption of turmeric)
- A slice of lemon or a dash of lemon juice (optional, for a refreshing twist and vitamin C)

Preparation time:	Cook time:	Total time:
5 min	10 min	15 min

DIRECTIONS

Simmer: In a small saucepan, bring the water or almond milk to a gentle simmer over medium heat. Add the grated turmeric, grated ginger, black pepper, and cinnamon stick. If using turmeric powder and ground cinnamon, whisk them in to ensure no lumps form.

Low Heat Infusion: Reduce the heat to low and let the mixture simmer gently for about 10 minutes. This allows the flavors and properties of the herbs to infuse into the liquid.

Strain: Remove the saucepan from the heat. Strain the tea through a fine mesh sieve into cups to remove the solid pieces of herbs and spices.

Add Sweetener and Oil: Stir in honey or maple syrup, if using, and coconut oil. Both add flavor and enhance the tea's health benefits. Coconut oil is essential if you aim to maximize curcumin's absorption.

Lemon Juice: Squeeze a slice of lemon into each cup or add a dash of lemon juice for an extra layer of flavor and a boost of vitamin C.

Serve and Enjoy: Serve the tea warm.

Nutritional Breakdown (Estimated per serving): Calories: 25 kcal (without optional ingredients), Protein: 0.5 g, Fat: 0.5 g, Carbs: 4 g (Note: Adding honey, coconut oil, or almond milk will alter these values.)

CHAPTER 13: HOLIDAY COOKING

CHRISTMAS STUFFED MUSHROOMS

INGREDIENTS

- 12 large cremini or button mushrooms, stems removed and finely chopped (reserve caps)
- 2 tablespoons olive oil, divided
- 1 small onion, finely chopped
- 2 cloves garlic, minced
- 1 cup spinach, chopped
- 1/2 cup quinoa, cooked
- 1/4 teaspoon turmeric
- 1/2 teaspoon smoked paprika
- Salt and pepper, to taste
- 2/4 cup dairy-free cheese
- Fresh parsley, chopped (for garnish)

Nutritional Breakdown (Estimated per serving):
Calories: 150 kcal, Protein: 6 g, Fat: 10 g (Saturated Fat: 1.5 g), Carbs: 12 g (Dietary Fiber: 3 g, Sugars: 4 g)

Preparation time:	Cook time:	Total time:
20 min	20 min	40 min

DIRECTIONS

Preheat Oven: Preheat your oven to 375°F (190°C). Line a baking sheet with parchment paper.

Sauté Vegetables: In a skillet over medium heat, heat 1 tablespoon of olive oil. Add the chopped mushroom stems, onion, and garlic. Sauté until the vegetables are soft and lightly browned, about 5-7 minutes.

Add Spinach and Spices: Stir in the chopped spinach, cooking until wilted. Add the cooked quinoa, turmeric, smoked paprika, salt, and pepper. Cook for another 2-3 minutes, stirring frequently.

Prepare Mushroom Caps: Brush the mushroom caps with the remaining olive oil and place them on the prepared baking sheet, stem-side up.

Stuff Mushrooms: Spoon the vegetable and quinoa mixture into the mushroom caps, pressing gently to fill them.

Bake: Bake in the preheated oven for 15-20 minutes or until the mushrooms are tender and the tops are lightly golden.

Garnish and Serve: Sprinkle the stuffed mushrooms with the dairy-free cheese and garnish with fresh parsley before serving.

CHRISTMAS ROASTED CHICKEN

INGREDIENTS
- 1 whole chicken (about 4-5 lbs)
- 2 tablespoons olive oil
- 1 teaspoon ground turmeric
- 2 teaspoons smoked paprika
- 1 teaspoon garlic powder
- 1/2 teaspoon ground ginger
- 1/2 teaspoon ground cinnamon
- Salt and pepper to taste
- 1 orange, quartered (for added moisture and a hint of sweetness)
- A handful of fresh herbs (thyme, rosemary, and parsley) for stuffing
- 2 tablespoons honey (optional, for a slight sweetness)
- Additional fresh herbs for garnish

Preparation time:	Cook time:	Total time:
20 min	1h 30 min	1 h 50 min

DIRECTIONS
Preheat Oven: Preheat your oven to 375°F (190°C).
Prepare the Chicken: Rinse the chicken under cold water and pat dry with paper towels. Place it in a roasting pan.
Mix the Spices: In a small bowl, combine the olive oil, turmeric, smoked paprika, garlic powder, ginger, cinnamon, salt, and pepper to form a paste.
Season the Chicken: Rub the spice paste evenly over the entire surface of the chicken, including under the skin, for deeper flavor penetration. If using honey, brush it over the chicken now for a caramelized glaze.
Stuff the Chicken: Stuff the cavity of the chicken with the quartered orange and a handful of fresh herbs.
Roast: Place the chicken in the preheated oven and roast for about 1 hour and 30 minutes, or until the juices run clear when the thickest part of the thigh is pierced with a skewer and the internal temperature reaches 165°F (74°C).
Rest: Remove the chicken from the oven and let it rest for 10 minutes before carving. This redistributes the juices, making the chicken moist and flavorful.
Garnish and Serve: Garnish the roasted chicken with additional fresh herbs before serving.

Nutritional Breakdown (Estimated per serving): Calories: 350 kcal, Protein: 25 g, Fat: 25 g (Saturated Fat: 5 g), Carbs: 5 g (Dietary Fiber: 1 g, Sugars: 2 g)

CHRISTMAS GINGER COOKIES

INGREDIENTS

- 2 cups gluten-free flour
- 1/4 cup coconut oil, melted
- 1/4 cup pure maple syrup (a natural sweetener)
- 1 teaspoon ground ginger
- 1/2 teaspoon ground cinnamon
- 1/4 teaspoon ground turmeric
- 1/4 teaspoon ground cloves
- 1/4 teaspoon fine sea salt
- 1/2 teaspoon baking soda
- 1 teaspoon vanilla extract

Nutritional Breakdown (Estimated per serving - 1 cookie): Calories: 90 kcal, Protein: 1 g, Fat: 4 g (Saturated Fat: 0.5 g), Carbs: 13 g (Dietary Fiber: 1 g, Sugars: 6 g)

Preparation time:	Cook time:	Total time:
15 min	10 min	25 min +chilling time

DIRECTIONS

Combine Dry Ingredients: In a large mixing bowl, whisk together the gluten-free flour, ground ginger, cinnamon, turmeric, cloves, sea salt, and baking soda.

Mix Wet Ingredients: In a separate bowl, mix the melted coconut oil, maple syrup, and vanilla extract until well combined.

Combine Wet and Dry Ingredients: Pour the wet ingredients into the dry ingredients and stir until a dough forms. The dough should be firm enough to handle; if it's too sticky, add a little more gluten-free flour.

Chill the Dough: Wrap the dough in plastic wrap and refrigerate for at least 30 minutes. This makes the dough easier to handle and helps the cookies hold their shape.

Preheat Oven: Preheat your oven to 350°F (175°C) and line a baking sheet with parchment paper.

Form Cookies: Once chilled, roll the dough into 1-inch balls and place them on the prepared baking sheet. Flatten each ball slightly with your palm or the bottom of a glass. If desired, use cookie cutters to create festive shapes.

Bake: Bake in the preheated oven for 8-10 minutes or until the edges are slightly golden. Be careful not to overbake.

Cool: Allow the cookies to cool on the baking sheet for 5 minutes before transferring them to a wire rack to cool completely.

Enjoy: These anti-inflammatory Christmas ginger cookies are perfect for holiday gatherings, offering a healthier alternative to traditional sugary treats.

THANKSGIVING STUFFED TURKEY

INGREDIENTS
- 1 whole turkey (10-12 lbs), thawed and ready to cook
- 1/4 cup olive oil
- 2 tablespoons ground turmeric
- 1 tablespoon ground ginger
- 2 teaspoons garlic powder
- 2 teaspoons smoked paprika
- Salt and pepper, to taste

For the Stuffing:
- 1 cup quinoa, cooked
- 1 large onion, diced
- 2 celery stalks, diced
- 1 apple, diced
- 1/2 cup dried cranberries
- 1/2 cup chopped walnuts (optional)
- 2 teaspoons fresh thyme, chopped
- 2 teaspoons fresh rosemary, chopped
- 2 tablespoons olive oil
- Salt and pepper, to taste

Nutritional Breakdown (Estimated per serving):
Calories: 450 kcal, Protein: 65 g, Fat: 20 g (Saturated Fat: 5 g), Carbs: 5 g (Dietary Fiber: 1 g, Sugars: 2 g)

Preparation time:	Cook time:	Total time:
30 min	3 h	3 h 30 min

DIRECTIONS
Preheat Oven: Preheat your oven to 325°F (165°C).

Prepare the Stuffing: In a large skillet, heat 2 tablespoons of olive oil over medium heat. Add the onion and celery, cooking until softened. Add the apple, dried cranberries, walnuts (if using), cooked quinoa, thyme, and rosemary. Season with salt and pepper. Cook for another 5 minutes, stirring occasionally. Remove from heat and let cool.

Prepare the Turkey: Pat the turkey dry with paper towels. In a small bowl, mix together the olive oil, turmeric, ginger, garlic powder, smoked paprika, salt, and pepper to form a paste. Rub this mixture under and over the turkey's skin, ensuring it is well-coated.

Stuff the Turkey: Once the stuffing has cooled, spoon it into the turkey's cavity. Tie the legs together with kitchen twine and tuck the wing tips under the body.

Roast the Turkey: Place the turkey breast-side up in a roasting pan. Tent the turkey with aluminum foil to prevent excessive browning. Roast in the preheated oven, calculating about 13 minutes of cooking time per pound. For a 10-12 lb turkey, this will be approximately 2.5 to 3 hours. Remove the foil in the last 45 minutes to make the skin golden and crispy.

Check for Doneness: The turkey is done when a meat thermometer inserted into the thickest part of the thigh reads 165°F (74°C).

Rest Before Carving: Let the turkey rest for at least 20 minutes before carving. This redistributes the juices, ensuring the meat is moist and flavorful.

Serve: Carve the turkey and serve with the stuffing and your favorite Thanksgiving sides.

THANKSGIVING BAKED SWEET POTATO

INGREDIENTS

- 4 medium sweet potatoes, scrubbed
- 2 tablespoons olive oil
- 1 teaspoon ground cinnamon
- 1/2 teaspoon ground turmeric
- 1/4 teaspoon ground ginger
- Salt and pepper to taste
- 1/4 cup pecans, roughly chopped (optional, for crunch)
- 2 tablespoons fresh parsley, finely chopped (for garnish)
- A drizzle of honey or maple syrup (optional for sweetness)

Preparation time:	Cook time:	Total time:
10 min	45-60 min	55-70 min

DIRECTIONS

Preheat Oven: Preheat your oven to 400°F (200°C). Line a baking sheet with parchment paper or aluminum foil for easy cleanup.

Prepare Sweet Potatoes: Pierce each sweet potato several times with a fork. This allows steam to escape during the baking process.

Season: Rub each sweet potato with olive oil, then sprinkle with cinnamon, turmeric, ginger, salt, and pepper. Place them on the prepared baking sheet.

Bake: Place the sweet potatoes in the preheated oven and bake for 45-60 minutes or until tender and fully cooked. The cooking time will vary depending on the size of the sweet potatoes.

Add Toppings: Split the sweet potatoes open with a knife once baked and slightly cooled. If desired, fluff the insides with a fork. Sprinkle with chopped pecans, parsley, and a drizzle of honey or maple syrup for added sweetness.

Serve: Serve the baked sweet potatoes warm as a nutritious and flavorful side dish that complements your Thanksgiving feast.

Serve: Carve the turkey and serve with the stuffing and your favorite Thanksgiving sides.

Nutritional Breakdown (Estimated per serving): Calories: 200 kcal, Protein: 2 g, Fat: 9 g (Saturated Fat: 1.3 g), Carbs: 28 g (Dietary Fiber: 4 g, Sugars: 7 g)

THANKSGIVING PUMPKIN SPICE MOUSSE

INGREDIENTS
- 1 can (15 oz) pure pumpkin puree
- 1 can (13.5 oz) full-fat coconut milk, chilled overnight
- 1/4 cup maple syrup, adjust to taste
- 1 teaspoon vanilla extract
- 1 teaspoon ground cinnamon
- 1/2 teaspoon ground ginger
- 1/4 teaspoon ground nutmeg
- 1/4 teaspoon ground turmeric
- Pinch of salt
- Optional toppings: chopped pecans, a sprinkle of cinnamon, or coconut whipped cream

Preparation time:	Chill time:	Total time:
15 min	2h	2 h 15 min

DIRECTIONS

Prepare Coconut Milk: Open the can of chilled coconut milk and scoop out the solid cream into a large mixing bowl, leaving the liquid behind (you can save the liquid for smoothies).

Whip Coconut Cream: Using an electric mixer, whip the coconut cream until light and fluffy, about 3-5 minutes.

Mix in Pumpkin and Spices: Add the pumpkin puree, maple syrup, vanilla extract, cinnamon, ginger, nutmeg, turmeric, and a pinch of salt to the whipped coconut cream. Beat until well combined and smooth.

Chill: Divide the mousse into serving dishes and chill in the refrigerator for at least 2 hours to set. The mousse will thicken, and the flavors will meld together during this time.

Serve: Once chilled and set, garnish the pumpkin spice mousse with your choice of toppings, such as chopped pecans, an extra sprinkle of cinnamon, or a dollop of coconut whipped cream.

Nutritional Breakdown (Estimated per serving): Calories: 180 kcal, Protein: 3 g, Fat: 14 g (Saturated Fat: 7 g), Carbs: 12 g (Dietary Fiber: 2 g, Sugars: 8 g)

CHAPTER 14: SAUCES

BEETROOT AND GINGER SAUCE

INGREDIENTS
- 2 medium beetroots, roasted and peeled
- 1 inch ginger, grated
- 2 tablespoons apple cider vinegar
- 1 tablespoon olive oil
- 1 teaspoon honey (optional for sweetness)
- Salt and pepper to taste
- Water or vegetable broth (as needed for consistency)

Preparation time:	Cook time:	Total time:
10 min	30 min	40 min

DIRECTIONS
Prepare Beetroots: Wrap beetroots in foil and roast in a preheated oven at 400°F (200°C) for about 30 minutes or until tender. Let cool, peel, and chop.
Blend Ingredients: In a blender, combine the roasted beetroots, grated ginger, apple cider vinegar, olive oil, and honey. Blend until smooth.
Adjust Consistency: If the sauce is too thick, add water or vegetable broth to reach your desired consistency.
Season: Taste and adjust seasoning with salt and pepper.
Serve: This vibrant sauce is perfect for adding a sweet and tangy flavor to salads and roasted vegetables or as a dip for grilled chicken.

Nutritional Breakdown (Estimated per serving): Calories: 60 kcal, Protein: 1 g, Fat: 3.5 g (Saturated Fat: 0.5 g), Carbs: 7 g (Dietary Fiber: 2 g, Sugars: 4 g)

AVOCADO CILANTRO LIME SAUCE

INGREDIENTS
- 1 ripe avocado
- 1/4 cup fresh cilantro leaves
- Juice of 1 lime
- 1 clove garlic, minced
- 2 tablespoons olive oil
- Salt and pepper to taste
- Water (as needed to reach desired consistency)

Preparation time:	Cook time:	Total time:
10 min	10 min	20 min

DIRECTIONS
Blend Ingredients: In a blender or food processor, combine the avocado, cilantro leaves, lime juice, minced garlic, and olive oil. Blend until smooth.
Adjust Consistency: If the sauce is too thick, add water a tablespoon at a time until you reach your desired consistency.
Season: Taste and adjust seasoning with salt and pepper.

Nutritional Breakdown (Estimated per serving): Calories: 80 kcal, Protein: 1 g, Fat: 7 g (Saturated Fat: 1 g), Carbs: 5 g (Dietary Fiber: 3 g, Sugars: 1 g)

CARROT GINGER MISO SAUCE

INGREDIENTS
- 2 medium carrots, peeled and chopped
- 1-inch piece of fresh ginger, peeled and grated
- 2 tablespoons white miso paste
- 2 tablespoons rice vinegar
- 1 tablespoon sesame oil
- 1 teaspoon honey (optional, for a hint of sweetness)
- Water or vegetable broth, as needed for consistency

Preparation time:	Cook time:	Total time:
10 min	15 min	25 min

DIRECTIONS

Cook Carrots: Add the chopped carrots to boiling water in a small pot and cook until tender, about 10-15 minutes. Drain and let cool slightly.

Blend Ingredients: In a blender, combine the cooked carrots, grated ginger, miso paste, rice vinegar, sesame oil, and honey (if using). Blend until smooth.

Adjust Consistency: If the sauce is too thick, add water or vegetable broth a little at a time until you achieve the desired consistency.

Season: Taste and adjust seasoning, adding more miso or vinegar if needed for balance.

Serve: This sauce is perfect for drizzling over steamed or roasted vegetables, as a dressing for salads, or as a flavorful sauce for fish or tofu.

Nutritional Breakdown (Estimated per serving): Calories: 80 kcal, Protein: 2 g, Fat: 3.5 g (Saturated Fat: 0.5 g), Carbs: 11 g (Dietary Fiber: 2 g, Sugars: 6 g)

Part 3: 75-day Meal Plan and Health Journal

75-DAY MEAL PLAN

DAY 1
Breakfast: Sweet Potato Hash with Spinach and Eggs
Lunch: Lentil Stuffed Bell Peppers
Dinner: Baked Salmon with Avocado Salsa
Snack: Roasted Chickpeas with Rosemary and Sea Salt
Dessert: Cherry Sorbet
Drink: Pineapple and Turmeric Smoothie

DAY 2
Breakfast: Avocado Toast with Poached Egg
Lunch: Turmeric Chicken and Quinoa
Dinner: Veggie Stir-Fry
Snack: Sweet Potato Chips with Cinnamon and Paprika
Dessert: Banana Nut Oatmeal Cups
Drink: Ginger Lemon Honey Tea

DAY 3
Breakfast: Turmeric Ginger Oatmeal
Lunch: Lemon Garlic Baked Cod with Asparagus
Dinner: Kale and Quinoa Salad with Orange-Tahini Dressing
Snack: Avocado Hummus
Dessert: Raspberry Cobbler
Drink: Golden Turmeric Tea Recipe

DAY 4
Breakfast: Sweet Potato & Kale Hash
Lunch: Ginger Turmeric Chicken Stir-Fry
Dinner: Roasted Beet and Goat Cheese Salad
Snack: Roasted Spiced Cauliflower
Dessert: Vegan Apple Tart with Walnut Crust
Drink: Turmeric Ginger Smoothie

DAY 5
Breakfast: Smoked Salmon and Avocado Omelet
Lunch: Spicy Sweet Potato and Black Bean Chili
Dinner: Salmon Pasta with Sun-Dried Tomatoes
Snack: Zesty Lime and Cilantro Quinoa
Dessert: Ginger Spiced Cookies
Drink: Strawberry Banana Smoothie

DAY 6
Breakfast: Chia Seed Pudding with Mango
Lunch: Vegan Coconut Chickpea Curry
Dinner: Buddha Bowl
Snack: Garlic Roasted Brussels Sprouts
Dessert: Peach Galette
Drink: Raspberry Mango Peach Smoothie

DAY 7
Breakfast: Blueberry Almond Protein Pancakes
Lunch: Spicy Lentil and Sweet Potato Stew
Dinner: Ginger-Lime Tofu with Broccoli Stir-Fry
Snack: Grilled Asparagus with Lemon Zest
Dessert: Cherry Sorbet
Drink: Pineapple and Turmeric Smoothie

DAY 8
Breakfast: Sweet Potato Hash with Spinach and Eggs
Lunch: Turmeric Quinoa with Roasted Vegetables
Dinner: Spicy Black Bean and Sweet Potato Tacos
Snack: Roasted Chickpeas with Rosemary and Sea Salt
Dessert: Banana Nut Oatmeal Cups
Drink: Ginger Lemon Honey Tea

DAY 9
Breakfast: Avocado Toast with Poached Egg
Lunch: Mozzarella, Basil & Zucchini Frittata
Dinner: Zucchini Noodles with Avocado Pesto
Snack: Sweet Potato Chips with Cinnamon and Paprika
Dessert: Raspberry Cobbler
Drink: Golden Turmeric Tea Recipe

DAY 10
Breakfast: Turmeric Ginger Oatmeal
Lunch: Chickpea and Kale Salad with Lemon-Tahini Dressing
Dinner: Lentil Stuffed Bell Peppers
Snack: Avocado Hummus
Dessert: Vegan Apple Tart with Walnut Crust
Drink: Turmeric Ginger Smoothie

DAY 11
Breakfast: Sweet Potato & Kale Hash
Lunch: Spicy Black Bean and Sweet Potato Tacos
Dinner: Mozzarella, Basil & Zucchini Frittata
Snack: Roasted Spiced Cauliflower
Dessert: Peach Galette
Drink: Raspberry Mango Peach Smoothie

DAY 12
Breakfast: Smoked Salmon and Avocado Omelet
Lunch: Zucchini Noodles with Avocado Pesto
Dinner: Chickpea and Kale Salad with Lemon-Tahini Dressing
Snack: Zesty Lime and Cilantro Quinoa
Dessert: Cherry Sorbet
Drink: Pineapple and Turmeric Smoothie

DAY 13
Breakfast: Chia Seed Pudding with Mango
Lunch: Lentil Stuffed Bell Peppers
Dinner: Baked Salmon with Avocado Salsa
Snack: Garlic Roasted Brussels Sprouts
Dessert: Banana Nut Oatmeal Cups
Drink: Ginger Lemon Honey Tea

DAY14
Breakfast: Blueberry Almond Protein Pancakes
Lunch: Roasted Beet and Goat Cheese Salad
Dinner: Spicy Sweet Potato and Black Bean Chili
Snack: Grilled Asparagus with Lemon Zest
Dessert: Banana Nut Oatmeal Cups
Drink: Ginger Lemon Honey Tea

DAY 15
Breakfast: Sweet Potato Hash with Spinach and Eggs
Lunch: Salmon Pasta with Sun-Dried Tomatoes
Dinner: Vegan Coconut Chickpea Curry
Snack: Roasted Chickpeas with Rosemary and Sea Salt
Dessert: Raspberry Cobbler
Drink: Golden Turmeric Tea Recipe

DAY 16
Breakfast: Avocado Toast with Poached Egg
Lunch: Buddha Bowl
Dinner: Spicy Lentil and Sweet Potato Stew
Snack: Sweet Potato Chips with Cinnamon and Paprika
Dessert: Vegan Apple Tart with Walnut Crust
Drink: Turmeric Ginger Smoothie

DAY 17
Breakfast: Turmeric Ginger Oatmeal
Lunch: Ginger-Lime Tofu with Broccoli Stir-Fry
Dinner: Turmeric Quinoa with Roasted Vegetables
Snack: Avocado Hummus
Dessert: Ginger Spiced Cookies
Drink: Strawberry Banana Smoothie

DAY 18
Breakfast: Sweet Potato & Kale Hash
Lunch: Spicy Black Bean and Sweet Potato Tacos
Dinner: Mozzarella, Basil & Zucchini Frittata
Snack: Roasted Spiced Cauliflower
Dessert: Peach Galette
Drink: Raspberry Mango Peach Smoothie

DAY 19
Breakfast: Smoked Salmon and Avocado Omelet
Lunch: Zucchini Noodles with Avocado Pesto
Dinner: Chickpea and Kale Salad with Lemon-Tahini Dressing
Snack: Zesty Lime and Cilantro Quinoa
Dessert: Cherry Sorbet
Drink: Pineapple and Turmeric Smoothie

DAY 20
Breakfast: Chia Seed Pudding with Mango
Lunch: Lentil Stuffed Bell Peppers
Dinner: Baked Salmon with Avocado Salsa
Snack: Garlic Roasted Brussels Sprouts
Dessert: Banana Nut Oatmeal Cups
Drink: Ginger Lemon Honey Tea

DAY 21
Breakfast: Blueberry Almond Protein Pancakes
Lunch: Turmeric Chicken and Quinoa
Dinner: Veggie Stir-Fry
Snack: Grilled Asparagus with Lemon Zest
Dessert: Raspberry Cobbler
Drink: Golden Turmeric Tea Recipe

DAY 22
Breakfast: Sweet Potato Hash with Spinach and Eggs
Lunch: Lemon Garlic Baked Cod with Asparagus
Dinner: Kale and Quinoa Salad with Orange-Tahini Dressing
Snack: Roasted Chickpeas with Rosemary and Sea Salt
Dessert: Vegan Apple Tart with Walnut Crust
Drink: Turmeric Ginger Smoothie

DAY 23
Breakfast: Avocado Toast with Poached Egg
Lunch: Ginger Turmeric Chicken Stir-Fry
Dinner: Roasted Beet and Goat Cheese Salad
Snack: Sweet Potato Chips with Cinnamon and Paprika
Dessert: Ginger Spiced Cookies
Drink: Strawberry Banana Smoothie

DAY 24
Breakfast: Turmeric Ginger Oatmeal
Lunch: Spicy Sweet Potato and Black Bean Chili
Dinner: Salmon Pasta with Sun-Dried Tomatoes
Snack: Avocado Hummus
Dessert: Peach Galette
Drink: Raspberry Mango Peach Smoothie

DAY 25
Breakfast: Sweet Potato & Kale Hash
Lunch: Vegan Coconut Chickpea Curry
Dinner: Buddha Bowl
Snack: Roasted Spiced Cauliflower
Dessert: Cherry Sorbet
Drink: Pineapple and Turmeric Smoothie

DAY 26
Breakfast: Smoked Salmon and Avocado Omelet
Lunch: Spicy Lentil and Sweet Potato Stew
Dinner: Ginger-Lime Tofu with Broccoli Stir-Fry
Snack: Zesty Lime and Cilantro Quinoa
Dessert: Banana Nut Oatmeal Cups
Drink: Ginger Lemon Honey Tea

DAY 27
Breakfast: Chia Seed Pudding with Mango
Lunch: Turmeric Quinoa with Roasted Vegetables
Dinner: Spicy Black Bean and Sweet Potato Tacos
Snack: Garlic Roasted Brussels Sprouts
Dessert: Raspberry Cobbler
Drink: Golden Turmeric Tea

DAY 28
Breakfast: Smoked Salmon and Avocado Omelet
Lunch: Spicy Black Bean and Sweet Potato Tacos
Dinner: Mozzarella, Basil & Zucchini Frittata
Snack: Zesty Lime and Cilantro Quinoa
Dessert: Raspberry Cobbler
Drink: Golden Turmeric Tea Recipe

DAY 29
Breakfast: Sweet Potato Hash with Spinach and Eggs
Lunch: Chickpea and Kale Salad with Lemon-Tahini Dressing
Dinner: Lentil Stuffed Bell Peppers
Snack: Roasted Chickpeas with Rosemary and Sea Salt
Dessert: Ginger Spiced Cookies
Drink: Strawberry Banana Smoothie

DAY 30
Breakfast: Avocado Toast with Poached Egg
Lunch: Baked Salmon with Avocado Salsa
Dinner: Turmeric Chicken and Quinoa
Snack: Sweet Potato Chips with Cinnamon and Paprika
Dessert: Peach Galette
Drink: Raspberry Mango Peach Smoothie

DAY 31
Breakfast: Turmeric Ginger Oatmeal
Lunch: Veggie Stir-Fry
Dinner: Lemon Garlic Baked Cod with Asparagus
Snack: Avocado Hummus
Dessert: Cherry Sorbet
Drink: Pineapple and Turmeric Smoothie

DAY 32
Breakfast: Sweet Potato & Kale Hash
Lunch: Kale and Quinoa Salad with Orange-Tahini Dressing
Dinner: Ginger Turmeric Chicken Stir-Fry
Snack: Roasted Spiced Cauliflower
Dessert: Banana Nut Oatmeal Cups
Drink: Ginger Lemon Honey Tea

DAY 33
Breakfast: Smoked Salmon and Avocado Omelet
Lunch: Roasted Beet and Goat Cheese Salad
Dinner: Spicy Sweet Potato and Black Bean Chili
Snack: Zesty Lime and Cilantro Quinoa
Dessert: Raspberry Cobbler
Drink: Golden Turmeric Tea Recipe

DAY 34
Breakfast: Chia Seed Pudding with Mango
Lunch: Salmon Pasta with Sun-Dried Tomatoes
Dinner: Vegan Coconut Chickpea Curry
Snack: Garlic Roasted Brussels Sprouts
Dessert: Vegan Apple Tart with Walnut Crust
Drink: Turmeric Ginger Smoothie

DAY 35
Breakfast: Blueberry Almond Protein Pancakes
Lunch: Buddha Bowl
Dinner: Spicy Lentil and Sweet Potato Stew
Snack: Grilled Asparagus with Lemon Zest
Dessert: Ginger Spiced Cookies
Drink: Strawberry Banana Smoothie

DAY 36
Breakfast: Sweet Potato Hash with Spinach and Eggs
Lunch: Ginger-Lime Tofu with Broccoli Stir-Fry
Dinner: Turmeric Quinoa with Roasted Vegetables
Snack: Roasted Chickpeas with Rosemary and Sea Salt
Dessert: Peach Galette
Drink: Raspberry Mango Peach Smooth

DAY 37
Breakfast: Avocado Toast with Poached Egg
Lunch: Spicy Black Bean and Sweet Potato Tacos
Dinner: Mozzarella, Basil & Zucchini Frittata
Snack: Sweet Potato Chips with Cinnamon and Paprika
Dessert: Cherry Sorbet
Drink: Pineapple and Turmeric Smoothie

DAY 38
Breakfast: Turmeric Ginger Oatmeal
Lunch: Zucchini Noodles with Avocado Pesto
Dinner: Chickpea and Kale Salad with Lemon-Tahini Dressing
Snack: Avocado Hummus
Dessert: Banana Nut Oatmeal Cups
Drink: Ginger Lemon Honey Tea

DAY 39
Breakfast: Sweet Potato & Kale Hash
Lunch: Lentil Stuffed Bell Peppers
Dinner: Baked Salmon with Avocado Salsa
Snack: Roasted Spiced Cauliflower
Dessert: Raspberry Cobbler
Drink: Golden Turmeric Tea Recipe
DAY 40

Breakfast: Smoked Salmon and Avocado Omelet
Lunch: Turmeric Chicken and Quinoa
Dinner: Veggie Stir-Fry
Snack: Zesty Lime and Cilantro Quinoa
Dessert: Vegan Apple Tart with Walnut Crust
Drink: Turmeric Ginger Smoothie

DAY 41
Breakfast: Chia Seed Pudding with Mango
Lunch: Lemon Garlic Baked Cod with Asparagus
Dinner: Kale and Quinoa Salad with Orange-Tahini Dressing
Snack: Garlic Roasted Brussels Sprouts
Dessert: Ginger Spiced Cookies
Drink: Strawberry Banana Smoothie

DAY 42
Breakfast: Blueberry Almond Protein Pancakes
Lunch: Ginger Turmeric Chicken Stir-Fry
Dinner: Roasted Beet and Goat Cheese Salad
Snack: Grilled Asparagus with Lemon Zest
Dessert: Peach Galette
Drink: Raspberry Mango Peach Smoothie

DAY 43
Breakfast: Sweet Potato Hash with Spinach and Eggs
Lunch: Spicy Sweet Potato and Black Bean Chili
Dinner: Salmon Pasta with Sun-Dried Tomatoes
Snack: Roasted Chickpeas with Rosemary and Sea Salt
Dessert: Cherry Sorbet
Drink: Pineapple and Turmeric Smoothie

DAY 44
Breakfast: Avocado Toast with Poached Egg
Lunch: Vegan Coconut Chickpea Curry
Dinner: Buddha Bowl
Snack: Sweet Potato Chips with Cinnamon and Paprika
Dessert: Banana Nut Oatmeal Cups
Drink: Ginger Lemon Honey Tea

DAY 45
Breakfast: Turmeric Ginger Oatmeal
Lunch: Spicy Lentil and Sweet Potato Stew
Dinner: Ginger-Lime Tofu with Broccoli Stir-Fry
Snack: Avocado Hummus
Dessert: Raspberry Cobbler
Drink: Golden Turmeric Tea Recipe

DAY 46
Breakfast: Sweet Potato & Kale Hash
Lunch: Turmeric Quinoa with Roasted Vegetables
Dinner: Spicy Black Bean and Sweet Potato Tacos
Snack: Roasted Spiced Cauliflower
Dessert: Vegan Apple Tart with Walnut Crust
Drink: Turmeric Ginger Smoothie
DAY 47

Breakfast: Smoked Salmon and Avocado Omelet
Lunch: Mozzarella, Basil & Zucchini Frittata
Dinner: Zucchini Noodles with Avocado Pesto
Snack: Zesty Lime and Cilantro Quinoa
Dessert: Ginger Spiced Cookies
Drink: Strawberry Banana Smoothie

DAY 48
Breakfast: Chia Seed Pudding with Mango
Lunch: Chickpea and Kale Salad with Lemon-Tahini Dressing
Dinner: Lentil Stuffed Bell Peppers
Snack: Garlic Roasted Brussels Sprouts
Dessert: Peach Galette
Drink: Raspberry Mango Peach Smoothie

DAY 49
Breakfast: Blueberry Almond Protein Pancakes
Lunch: Baked Salmon with Avocado Salsa
Dinner: Turmeric Chicken and Quinoa
Snack: Grilled Asparagus with Lemon Zest
Dessert: Cherry Sorbet
Drink: Pineapple and Turmeric Smoothie

DAY 50
Breakfast: Sweet Potato Hash with Spinach and Eggs
Lunch: Veggie Stir-Fry
Dinner: Lemon Garlic Baked Cod with Asparagus
Snack: Roasted Chickpeas with Rosemary and Sea Salt
Dessert: Banana Nut Oatmeal Cups
Drink: Ginger Lemon Honey Tea
DAY 51

Breakfast: Avocado Toast with Poached Egg
Lunch: Kale and Quinoa Salad with Orange-Tahini Dressing
Dinner: Ginger Turmeric Chicken Stir-Fry
Snack: Sweet Potato Chips with Cinnamon and Paprika
Dessert: Raspberry Cobbler
Drink: Golden Turmeric Tea Recipe

DAY 52
Breakfast: Turmeric Ginger Oatmeal
Lunch: Roasted Beet and Goat Cheese Salad
Dinner: Spicy Sweet Potato and Black Bean Chili
Snack: Avocado Hummus
Dessert: Vegan Apple Tart with Walnut Crust
Drink: Turmeric Ginger Smoothie

DAY 53
Breakfast: Sweet Potato & Kale Hash
Lunch: Salmon Pasta with Sun-Dried Tomatoes
Dinner: Vegan Coconut Chickpea Curry
Snack: Roasted Spiced Cauliflower
Dessert: Ginger Spiced Cookies
Drink: Strawberry Banana Smoothie

DAY 54
Breakfast: Smoked Salmon and Avocado Omelet
Lunch: Buddha Bowl
Dinner: Spicy Lentil and Sweet Potato Stew
Snack: Zesty Lime and Cilantro Quinoa
Dessert: Peach Galette
Drink: Raspberry Mango Peach Smoothie

DAY 55
Breakfast: Chia Seed Pudding with Mango
Lunch: Ginger-Lime Tofu with Broccoli Stir-Fry
Dinner: Turmeric Quinoa with Roasted Vegetables
Snack: Garlic Roasted Brussels Sprouts
Dessert: Cherry Sorbet
Drink: Pineapple and Turmeric Smoothie

DAY 56
Breakfast: Blueberry Almond Protein Pancakes
Lunch: Spicy Black Bean and Sweet Potato Tacos
Dinner: Mozzarella, Basil & Zucchini Frittata
Snack: Grilled Asparagus with Lemon Zest
Dessert: Banana Nut Oatmeal Cups
Drink: Ginger Lemon Honey Tea

DAY 57
Breakfast: Sweet Potato Hash with Spinach and Eggs
Lunch: Zucchini Noodles with Avocado Pesto
Dinner: Chickpea and Kale Salad with Lemon-Tahini Dressing
Snack: Roasted Chickpeas with Rosemary and Sea Salt
Dessert: Raspberry Cobbler
Drink: Golden Turmeric Tea Recipe

DAY 58
Breakfast: Avocado Toast with Poached Egg
Lunch: Lentil Stuffed Bell Peppers
Dinner: Baked Salmon with Avocado Salsa
Snack: Sweet Potato Chips with Cinnamon and Paprika
Dessert: Vegan Apple Tart with Walnut Crust
Drink: Turmeric Ginger Smoothie

DAY 59
Breakfast: Turmeric Ginger Oatmeal
Lunch: Turmeric Chicken and Quinoa
Dinner: Veggie Stir-Fry
Snack: Avocado Hummus
Dessert: Ginger Spiced Cookies
Drink: Strawberry Banana Smoothie

DAY 60
Breakfast: Sweet Potato & Kale Hash
Lunch: Lemon Garlic Baked Cod with Asparagus
Dinner: Kale and Quinoa Salad with Orange-Tahini Dressing
Snack: Roasted Spiced Cauliflower
Dessert: Peach Galette
Drink: Raspberry Mango Peach Smoothie

DAY 61
Breakfast: Smoked Salmon and Avocado Omelet
Lunch: Ginger Turmeric Chicken Stir-Fry
Dinner: Roasted Beet and Goat Cheese Salad
Snack: Zesty Lime and Cilantro Quinoa
Dessert: Cherry Sorbet
Drink: Pineapple and Turmeric Smoothie

DAY 62
Breakfast: Chia Seed Pudding with Mango
Lunch: Spicy Sweet Potato and Black Bean Chili
Dinner: Salmon Pasta with Sun-Dried Tomatoes
Snack: Garlic Roasted Brussels Sprouts
Dessert: Banana Nut Oatmeal Cups
Drink: Ginger Lemon Honey Tea

DAY 63
Breakfast: Blueberry Almond Protein Pancakes
Lunch: Vegan Coconut Chickpea Curry
Dinner: Buddha Bowl
Snack: Grilled Asparagus with Lemon Zest
Dessert: Raspberry Cobbler
Drink: Golden Turmeric Tea Recipe

DAY 64
Breakfast: Sweet Potato Hash with Spinach and Eggs
Lunch: Spicy Lentil and Sweet Potato Stew
Dinner: Ginger-Lime Tofu with Broccoli Stir-Fry
Snack: Roasted Chickpeas with Rosemary and Sea Salt
Dessert: Vegan Apple Tart with Walnut Crust
Drink: Turmeric Ginger Smoothie

DAY 65
Breakfast: Avocado Toast with Poached Egg
Lunch: Turmeric Quinoa with Roasted Vegetables
Dinner: Spicy Black Bean and Sweet Potato Tacos
Snack: Sweet Potato Chips with Cinnamon and Paprika
Dessert: Ginger Spiced Cookies
Drink: Strawberry Banana Smoothie

DAY 66
Breakfast: Turmeric Ginger Oatmeal
Lunch: Mozzarella, Basil & Zucchini Frittata
Dinner: Zucchini Noodles with Avocado Pesto
Snack: Avocado Hummus
Dessert: Peach Galette
Drink: Raspberry Mango Peach Smoothie

DAY 67
Breakfast: Sweet Potato & Kale Hash
Lunch: Chickpea and Kale Salad with Lemon-Tahini Dressing
Dinner: Lentil Stuffed Bell Peppers
Snack: Roasted Spiced Cauliflower
Dessert: Cherry Sorbet
Drink: Pineapple and Turmeric Smoothie

DAY 68
Breakfast: Smoked Salmon and Avocado Omelet
Lunch: Baked Salmon with Avocado Salsa
Dinner: Turmeric Chicken and Quinoa
Snack: Zesty Lime and Cilantro Quinoa
Dessert: Banana Nut Oatmeal Cups
Drink: Ginger Lemon Honey Tea

DAY 69
Breakfast: Chia Seed Pudding with Mango
Lunch: Veggie Stir-Fry
Dinner: Lemon Garlic Baked Cod with Asparagus
Snack: Garlic Roasted Brussels Sprouts
Dessert: Raspberry Cobbler
Drink: Golden Turmeric Tea Recipe

DAY 70
Breakfast: Blueberry Almond Protein Pancakes
Lunch: Kale and Quinoa Salad with Orange-Tahini Dressing
Dinner: Ginger Turmeric Chicken Stir-Fry
Snack: Grilled Asparagus with Lemon Zest
Dessert: Vegan Apple Tart with Walnut Crust
Drink: Turmeric Ginger Smoothie

DAY 71
Breakfast: Sweet Potato Hash with Spinach and Eggs
Lunch: Roasted Beet and Goat Cheese Salad
Dinner: Spicy Sweet Potato and Black Bean Chili
Snack: Roasted Chickpeas with Rosemary and Sea Salt
Dessert: Ginger Spiced Cookies
Drink: Strawberry Banana Smoothie

DAY 72
Breakfast: Avocado Toast with Poached Egg
Lunch: Salmon Pasta with Sun-Dried Tomatoes
Dinner: Vegan Coconut Chickpea Curry
Snack: Sweet Potato Chips with Cinnamon and Paprika
Dessert: Peach Galette
Drink: Raspberry Mango Peach Smoothie

DAY 73
Breakfast: Turmeric Ginger Oatmeal
Lunch: Buddha Bowl
Dinner: Spicy Lentil and Sweet Potato Stew
Snack: Avocado Hummus
Dessert: Cherry Sorbet
Drink: Pineapple and Turmeric Smoothie

DAY 74
Breakfast: Sweet Potato & Kale Hash
Lunch: Ginger-Lime Tofu with Broccoli Stir-Fry
Dinner: Turmeric Quinoa with Roasted Vegetables
Snack: Roasted Spiced Cauliflower
Dessert: Banana Nut Oatmeal Cups
Drink: Ginger Lemon Honey Tea

DAY 75
Breakfast: Smoked Salmon and Avocado Omelet
Lunch: Spicy Black Bean and Sweet Potato Tacos
Dinner: Mozzarella, Basil & Zucchini Frittata
Snack: Zesty Lime and Cilantro Quinoa
Dessert: Raspberry Cobbler
Drink: Golden Turmeric Tea Recipe

THE HEALTH JOURNAL

Welcome to your personal health journal, designed to guide you through an anti-inflammatory lifestyle. This journal is more than just a place to record your meals and workouts; it's a comprehensive tool to help you set intentions, track your progress, and reflect on your journey toward optimal health.

Beginning Your Journey: Setting Intentions and Goals

The journey to reducing inflammation and enhancing wellness begins with clarity. This section is dedicated to helping you articulate clear, achievable goals and intentions for your anti-inflammatory lifestyle.

How to Use:
- **Reflect**: Begin by reflecting on your current health status and what you hope to achieve by adopting an anti-inflammatory lifestyle. Are you looking to reduce symptoms, enhance energy, or improve overall well-being?
- **Set Goals**: Write down specific, measurable, achievable, relevant, and time-bound (SMART) goals. For example, "Reduce joint pain from a 7 to a 3 on the pain scale within three months."
- **Declare Intentions**: Beyond specific goals, set broader intentions for your journey, such as "Embrace a more plant-based diet" or "Cultivate mindfulness around eating."

Reflecting on Your Why

Ask yourself:

- What health concerns am I hoping to address through this lifestyle?
- How do I envision my life improving as I reduce inflammation?
- What personal milestones do I wish to achieve (e.g., increased energy, reduced pain)?

Document your reflections in detail, allowing them to guide your goal-setting process.

Crafting SMART Goals

Setting SMART (Specific, Measurable, Achievable, Relevant, Time-bound) goals transforms your aspirations into actionable steps. For each goal, consider:

- **Specific**: Define what success looks like. Instead of "eat healthier," aim for "incorporate two servings of anti-inflammatory vegetables into each meal."

- **Measurable**: Ensure you can track your progress. If your goal is to improve gut health, you might track the diversity of plant-based foods consumed weekly.
- **Achievable**: Set goals that challenge you without setting the bar too high. Consider your current lifestyle and what adjustments are realistic for you.
- **Relevant**: Align your goals with your broader health objectives and motivations. Each goal should be a building block toward your ultimate vision of wellness.
- **Time-bound**: Attach a timeframe to each goal. Whether it's three months to lower your CRP levels or two weeks to establish a daily meditation practice, deadlines create urgency and focus.

Establishing Intentions

While goals are your destinations, intentions are the mindset and values that will guide your daily actions and decisions. They are broader and help frame your journey in a positive, growth-oriented light. Set intentions such as:

- To approach my dietary choices with curiosity and openness, exploring new foods and flavors.
- To listen to my body's signals with compassion, understanding that healing is not linear.
- To cultivate patience and kindness towards myself, recognizing that every small step forward is progress.

Visualizing Success

Take a moment to visualize what achieving your goals and living according to your intentions will look like. Imagine how you will feel, the activities you'll enjoy, and the impact on your relationships and daily life. This visualization exercise can be a powerful motivator, especially on days when the path seems challenging.

Regular Review and Reflection

Finally, commit to regularly reviewing your goals and intentions. Life changes, and so will your needs and priorities. Set monthly check-ins to reflect on your progress, celebrate your victories, and adjust your course as needed. This dynamic approach ensures your anti-inflammatory journey remains aligned with your evolving wellness vision.

Daily Nourishment Log: Tracking Your Anti-Inflammatory Foods

Keeping a detailed food diary is about more than just accountability: it's a way to intimately understand how different foods impact your body, mood, and inflammation levels. By recording your meals, you can:

- Identify patterns and correlations between your diet and symptoms of inflammation or well-being.
- Discover which foods energize you and which ones may trigger negative responses.
- Gradually tailor a diet that suits your unique bio-individuality, maximizing anti-inflammatory benefits.

How to Track Effectively

- **Be Specific**: Record everything you eat and drink, including portion sizes and preparation methods.
- **Note the Time and Setting**: Sometimes, when and where we eat can affect how our bodies respond to food. Jot down the time of your meals and snacks, as well as any notable details about the setting.
- **Monitor Symptoms**: Alongside your food entries, note any physical or emotional symptoms you experience. This could include digestive discomfort, changes in energy levels, mood fluctuations, or joint pain. Over time, you may start to see patterns that link certain foods with specific symptoms.
- **Include Anti-Inflammatory Heroes**: Make a special note of foods known for their anti-inflammatory properties that you incorporate into your diet.
- **Reflect on Your Appetite and Fullness**: Pay attention to your hunger cues and how satisfied you feel after meals.

To truly benefit from your Daily Nourishment Log, consistency is key. Try to make logging as seamless as possible. Remember, the goal of the Daily Nourishment Log isn't to judge or restrict yourself but to cultivate a deeper understanding and appreciation of how food influences your health and well-being. It's a tool to empower you to make informed choices, celebrate dietary diversity, and ultimately, craft a personalized anti-inflammatory diet that supports your health goals.

Symptom and Wellness Tracker: Tuning into Your Body

Our bodies communicate with us constantly, but in the hustle of daily life, these messages can be overlooked or misunderstood. By systematically tracking your symptoms and overall well-being, you create a detailed map of your health landscape. This map not only helps identify patterns and triggers but also illuminates the path to greater wellness.

Your Symptom and Wellness Tracker should be comprehensive yet manageable. Consider including the following categories:

- **Date and Time**: Note the date and, if relevant, time of day for each entry to help identify patterns.

- **Dietary Intake**: Briefly record what you ate. Pay particular attention to new foods or deviations from your typical diet.
- **Symptoms**: List any physical or emotional symptoms you experience. This can range from joint pain and digestive discomfort to mood swings and energy levels.
- **Severity**: Rate the severity of your symptoms on a scale (e.g., 1-10). This helps track fluctuations over time.
- **Activity Level**: Note your physical activity, including type, duration, and intensity. Physical activity can influence inflammation and overall well-being.
- **Sleep Quality**: Record the quantity and quality of your sleep, as sleep significantly impacts inflammation and health.
- **Stress Levels**: Note your stress levels and any significant stressors. Stress is a known contributor to inflammation.
- **Overall Well-Being**: End each entry with a general assessment of your well-being. This holistic view helps contextualize the specific details recorded earlier.

Analyzing Your Data

Over time, your Symptom and Wellness Tracker will accumulate a wealth of data. Regularly review your entries to identify trends:

- **Food Reactions**: Are certain foods consistently followed by adverse symptoms?
- **Time Patterns**: Do symptoms emerge at specific times of day or week?
- **Activity Impact**: How does physical activity affect your symptoms and overall well-being?
- **Stress Correlation**: Is there a link between your stress levels and symptom severity?
- **Sleep Connection**: Observe how changes in sleep patterns influence your symptoms and mood.

Armed with insights from your tracker, you can begin to make targeted adjustments to your lifestyle by eliminating or reducing foods that seem to exacerbate symptoms, tailoring your exercise routine to balance activity with rest, implementing stress-reduction techniques that show promise in lowering your stress markers, and adjusting your evening routine to improve sleep quality and duration, based on your observations.

Mindful Eating Reflections: Cultivating Awareness and Gratitude

Mindful eating is an ancient practice that harmonizes body and mind, inviting full presence during meals. It's about engaging all your senses to truly experience the food on your plate. This conscious approach to eating can significantly improve digestion, reduce overeating, and enhance your emotional relationship with food.

Cultivating Mindfulness

Begin by setting the scene for a mindful meal, free from the distractions of technology or work. As you sit down to eat, take a few deep breaths to center yourself in the present moment.

- **Visual Appreciation**: Observe the colors and textures on your plate. Appreciate the journey each ingredient took to reach you.
- **Aromatic Anticipation**: Inhale deeply, taking in the aromas. Anticipation heightens the eventual taste experience.
- **Tactile Connection**: Notice the utensils in your hand, the texture of the food as you prepare to take a bite. Even this has a story.
- **Savoring Each Bite**: Chew slowly, allowing the flavors to unfold. Identify the individual taste notes and how they combine to create a harmonious dish.
- **Reflecting on the Nutritional Value**: As you eat, consider the nutrients entering your body, feeding your cells, and supporting your anti-inflammatory efforts.

With each meal, take a moment to express gratitude—not just for the food, but for the hands that prepared it, the earth that grew it, and the circumstances that brought it to you. This gratitude can transform your meal into an act of joyful celebration and a reminder of your connection to the world around you.

After each meal, jot down a few lines about the experience. What did you notice that was new or different? How did the act of eating mindfully make you feel?

Be thankful for the diversity of anti-inflammatory foods available to you, recognizing the abundance that allows you to eat such a health-promoting diet.

As you practice mindful eating and gratitude, you might notice a ripple effect in other areas of your life. This heightened awareness can lead to a more profound appreciation for your body's capabilities, the progress you're making on your anti-inflammatory path, and the simple pleasures that each day holds.

Physical Activity and Movement Diary: Complementing Your Diet with Exercise

Physical activity is a powerful ally in the battle against inflammation. Regular movement helps to moderate the body's inflammatory response, promoting the release of anti-inflammatory chemicals and reducing stress hormones that can exacerbate inflammation.

How to Use Your Movement Diary

- **Daily Activity Log**: Record your physical activities each day, noting the type (e.g., walking, swimming, resistance training), duration, and intensity level.
- **Body Responses**: Pay attention to how your body feels during and after exercise. Do certain activities leave you feeling energized while others lead to unnecessary pain or fatigue?
- **Symptom Fluctuations**: Keep an eye on how your exercise habits influence your inflammation-related symptoms.
- **Inflammation Markers**: If you're tracking inflammation markers through blood tests, note any changes that correlate with changes in your exercise habits.
- **Rest and Recovery**: Don't forget to document your rest days. Recovery is when your body repairs and strengthens itself, which is just as important as the activity itself.

Over time, your diary will reveal trends and patterns. You might discover that moderate-intensity activities are your sweet spot or that your body prefers cycling over running. Use this data to refine your approach, gradually building an exercise program that feels good and supports your anti-inflammatory goals.

CONCLUSION

As you close the final pages of this journey through the world of anti-inflammatory living, you stand at the threshold of a new beginning. You've traversed the landscape of inflammation, delved into the healing power of food, and personalized your diet to meet the unique needs of your body. You've explored an array of recipes that not only tantalize your taste buds but also serve to protect and heal your body from within.

You've learned that inflammation, while a natural defense mechanism, can sometimes linger like an unwelcome guest, and you now possess the knowledge to gently show it the door. From the complexities of chronic inflammation to the specific challenges it poses in conditions like rheumatoid arthritis and during life transitions such as menopause, you've discovered the connections that tie our gut health to our overall well-being and the profound impact that dietary choices can have on our body's inflammatory response. With each chapter, from the Omega-3 rich depths of the sea to the antioxidant-packed corners of the earth, you've been equipped with the tools to reduce inflammation through delicious, whole foods. You've debunked myths and learned to navigate social eating, all while understanding how bio-individuality shapes your unique path to health.

The recipes you've encountered are more than just meals; they are your allies in a quest for a life full of energy and devoid of unnecessary discomfort. The holiday treats and soothing teas are testaments to the fact that an anti-inflammatory diet can be both indulgent and healing.

As you move forward with your 75-day meal plan and continue to document your progress in your health journal, remember that this book is not just a guide but a companion. The goals and intentions you've set, the foods you've savored, and the activities you've logged are the threads weaving the tapestry of your health. You are now empowered to live vibrantly, with the wisdom to support your body in a way that reduces inflammation and enhances your quality of life.

As you continue this path, your journey is a story worth sharing If this book has found a special place in your kitchen and your heart, I invite you to leave a review on Amazon. Let your words be the bridge for someone else's journey to wellness. Share how the flavors and knowledge within these pages have changed your life, how they've brought joy to your table, and how they can promise the same transformation for countless others. Your insights and experiences are invaluable, and your review could be the guiding star for someone else on their journey to wellness.

So, if you have a moment, please leave a review on Amazon. Your words might just be the nudge someone else needs to embark on their own transformative journey. Let's spread the word and the health together.

Thank you for inviting this book into your kitchen, your heart, and your life. May your days be as flavor-filled as they are inflammation-free. Here's to a bright, healthful future and the many delicious moments to come.

Made in the USA
Monee, IL
13 September 2024

65763782R00070